MCQ Tutor In Anaesthesia: Part 1 FRCA

Colin A. Pinnock
MB BS FRCA
Consultant Anaesthetist, Alexandra Hospital, Redditch, UK

Robert P. Jones
MB ChB DA (UK)
Staff Anaesthetist, Alexandra Hospital, Redditch, UK

CHURCHILL LIVINGSTONE
EDINBURGH LONDON MADRID MELBOURNE NEW YORK AND TOKYO 1994

CHURCHILL LIVINGSTONE
Medical Division of Longman Group UK Limited

Distributed in the United States of America by Churchill
Livingstone Inc., 650 Avenue of the Americas, New York,
N.Y. 10011, and by associated companies, branches and
representatives throughout the world.

First published 1994

ISBN 0-443-04963-7

British Library Cataloguing in Publication Data
A catalogue record for this book is available from the British
Library.

Library of Congress Cataloging in Publication Data
A catalog record for this book is available from the
Library of Congress.

The
publisher's
policy is to use
paper manufactured
from sustainable forests

Produced by Longman Singapore Publishers Pte Ltd
Printed in Singapore

Contents

Preface

This volume completes the series of three MCQ revision textbooks designed to cover the examinations leading up to the FRCA diploma, although paradoxically it has been the last in the series to be written.

We have reproduced the format and style of questions as used in the examination. Each group of sixty questions can be used as an individual practice examination or the database of questions may be studied as a whole according to candidate preference.

We would suggest that the book is first used as a 'tutor' in the fashion described in the section 'How to Use the Book'. The technique of providing a specific answer for every completion with an individual reference to standard textbooks has proved popular in previous volumes and has thus been repeated. Readers can both satisfy themselves of the validity of the answer and read around the topics where necessary. The answers and referenced texts may also form the basis for discussion of a subject with mentors.

Questions have been carefully designed to closely mimic those which may appear in the Part 1 FRCA examination. The examination candidate may be confronted with imperfectly constructed questions and ambiguities that cannot be discussed on the answer sheet. Examples of this within the volume are highlighted for readers' benefit. Stems which are similar occur on occasions with different completions. This is deliberate and attempts to emulate the spread which may be found in reality, when in any one examination there may be more than one question on a particular topic. A few questions may be similar to those found in other revision texts; every effort has been taken to avoid such similarities which are unintentional.

Finally we would like to thank our colleagues at the Alexandra Hospital for their help and patience over the period of writing the series. Our special thanks are due to Dr Tracey Else for providing a 'candidate's eye view' of the manuscript.

Alexandra Hospital,   C.A. Pinnock
Redditch, 1993   R.P. Jones

A Guide to the Part 1 FRCA Examination

THE FRCA DIPLOMA

The three part examination for the Diploma of Fellow of the Royal College of Anaesthetists is intended to test both depth of knowledge and application of that knowledge across the fields of anaesthesia covered in basic specialist training (BST). In brief these comprise general anaesthetic practice, intensive care medicine and the relief of pain.

THE FRCA PART 1

The first part of the examination is designed to test the fundamentals of clinical practice. No recognised period of anaesthetic training is compulsory before sitting the Part 1 examination but the Royal College states that the examination is appropriate for the trainee who has reached the end of the first year of training in anaesthesia.

EXAMINATION STRUCTURE

The examination has four sections.

Sixty multiple choice questions of the stem and five completions (true/false) format. Time allowed – 2 hours

Seven compulsory written answers. Time allowed – 3 hours (held on the same day as the multiple choice paper).

Clinical oral using guided questions. The guided question consists of 10 minutes to study written information and test results e.g. ECG or X-ray on a hypothetical patient. There is then a 30 minute oral examination with two examiners.

Equipment and techniques oral. Designed to test physical principles and safe use af anaesthetic and monitoring equipment but anaesthetic techniques also come under scrutiny. Time allowed – 30 minutes with two examiners.

EXAMINATION CONTENT

No syllabus is issued for the examination but a guide to the content of the examination is issued by the Royal College of Anaesthetists. The goals of the examination are to test the candidates' knowledge of the following areas: administration of general and local anaesthetics to adults and children (excluding neonates), appropriate post-operative pain relief, immediate care and resuscitation (including advanced cardiopulmonary resuscitation), management of emergencies and stabilisation of patients and principles of obstetric anaesthesia and analgesia, physical principles underlying the function of equipment including monitoring and a knowledge of accuracy and limitations of equipment.

In addition candidates should be able to show an ability for recognizing the implications of medical and surgical disease in preoperative assessment, be conversant in anatomy of all areas relevant to local and general anaesthesia and understand the physiological principles and the pharmacology of processes and drugs that are encountered in anaesthetic practice.

EXAMINATION MARKING

The marking system used is described as a close-marking system. Each section of the examination (1 written, 1 MCQ and 2 oral sections) are given a mark. The marks used are as follows:

2 + A good pass, very difficult to obtain.
2   A pass.
1 + A fail by a very small margin.
1   A bad fail.

The marks required to pass the examination are 2, 2, 2, 1 + or better. There is no carry over between sections. Borderline candidates are discussed by the examiners before final results are issued.

THE DA (UK)

Success in FRCA Part 1 and proof of completion of a year in a schedule I or II hospital allows the candidate to apply for the diploma of DA (UK). This must be claimed within three years of passing the examination.

FURTHER INFORMATION

Detailed information on all parts of the examination is available in the Royal College publication entitled 'Guide to Training', May 1990. This is available on request from The Royal College of Anaesthetists, 48–49 Russell Square, London WC1B 4JP. Alternatively it can be obtained from local College Tutors. A detailed annual update can be found in the 'Handbook of British Anaesthesia' also available from the Royal College of Anaesthetists.

Notes on MCQ Technique

Multiple choice question papers are designed to test factual recall. Throughout the three parts of the FRCA the same multiple choice format is used. This consists of an interrogative or <u>stem</u> followed by five separate <u>completions</u> which may be marked true, false or don't know.

Candidates score +1 mark for each correct response and –1 for each incorrect response while 'don't know' scores zero. In the examination a question book is provided in which are the stems and completions and also a lector sheet on which to mark answer choices by way of pencilled bars. It is most strongly advised that answers are made in the question book before transferring them to the lector sheet. At this stage be absolutely scrupulous in marking the lector sheet in accordance with your answers as minor errors in numbering will prove disastrous. It is all too easy under stress to become confused.

Certain pitfalls deserve mention. Double check any question or part relating to opposites, for example hypo and hyper. If you get the sense reversed then minus five marks will result.

Beware of double negatives which needlessly confuse. While ideally there should not be any, in reality you will meet a few at least. Do not be overly suspicious of obvious false distractors. It is tempting to assume that if only you were more widely read then you would know of the connection between serum molybdenum and halothane hepatitis. Readers will be quick to spot that extensive reading is essential as a defence against this situation. Subjects which involve a great deal of controversy and debate may be best avoided for safety but there is an obvious limit to that particular gambit. There are remarkably few MCQ questions which are all true or all false but remember that these occasionally occur. Be very suspicious of 'always' and 'never' in a stem. It is also difficult to put value judgements on 'frequently' and 'often'.

In summary, practical points to keep in the front of your mind as you confront the question paper are listed overleaf for emphasis.

MOST IMPORTANT – DO NOT GUESS!

1. Read each question very carefully.
2. Make sure that you fully understand it.
3. Be especially wary of questions with opposites.
4. Do not spend too much time on any one question.
5. Think clearly and do not panic.
6. Do not pursue the answer too far but respond only to the simple question which has been posed.
7. Leave sufficient time to complete the lector sheet.

How to Use the Book

The maximum benefit from using this book as a revision aid will be obtained if the basic reading has been completed first. The layout of the book is consistent and questions are structured in five blocks of sixty. This deliberately mirrors the number in the present examination structure. As you work through the book you will find on the left-hand page three questions. Below them on the same page are listed the references which are keyed to the answers. Each triplet of questions has the answers displayed on the right-hand page.

It is suggested for revision that a sheet of paper or card is used to cover the answers while the questions are being attempted. Apart from concealing the answers this sheet may be used to record your choices for each completion. If a question is encountered about which you know very little, use the references below to read around the subject before answering. This will make the most of the revision exercise.

The references are quoted in shortened form and many of them will be familiar. A complete list, of the short references will be found in the bibliography at the back of the book. They are listed in full in alphabetical order and any unfamiliar source can be identified. Rather than being merely a list, the bibliography also gives some weight to the respective relevance of each text. Scanning it will indicate the scope of the reading necessary. All the texts are the currently available editions at the time of going to print. Occasional reference may have been made to an earlier edition out of necessity; this is marked as such in the short references.

Finally, there is an index of subjects at the end of the book. Where a topic in the index is followed by a number alone this indicates that the whole question is on that subject. In contrast, if a topic is followed by a number and a letter then it is the completion within a question which relates. For example, in the index 'Acetazolamide 242, 298b' indicates that Acetazolamide is the main subject and applies to all completions in question 242 and is featured in question 298 completion (b) only. The index will enable the selection of any one particular topic for revision by indicating each and every occasion on which that topic occurs.

---

1 Ketamine:
   a) may be given intrathecally
   b) stimulates respiration
   c) increases salivation
   d) may be given orally
   e) produces analgesia which is not reversed by naloxone

---

2 Features of fat embolism include:
   a) fat in the sputum
   b) fat in the urine
   c) petechial haemorrhages
   d) apyrexia
   e) eye changes

---

3 Halothane is associated with:
   a) potentiation of the action of D-tubocurarine
   b) a fall in skin temperature
   c) decreased renal blood flow
   d) increased serum bromide levels
   e) trifluoroacetic acid in the urine

References	
1.1 Synopsis	p 179–182
2.1 Synopsis	p 843–844
3.1 Synopsis	p 138–145

1a) T Ketamine has been used for spinal anaesthesia during war surgery but it is not specifically licensed for this use. Ketamine may also be given extradurally (1.1).

b) T Respiration is usually mildly stimulated. Respiratory depression is only observed after large doses of ketamine. Ketamine is a bronchodilator (1.1).

c) T Increased salivation occurs and may be controlled by the administration of atropine (1.1).

d) T Ketamine can be given orally, rectally, intravenously or intramuscularly and has been used for Bier's technique of intravenous regional anaesthesia (IVRA) (1.1).

e) F Ketamine analgesia is partially reversed by naloxone (1.1).

2a) T Fat can be seen in the sputum and urine on microscopy. The sputum is often frothy (2.1).

b) T Fat globules may be seen in the urine on microscopy (2.1).

c) T Petechial haemorrhages occur, with a purpuric eruption, over the upper chest, neck and conjunctivae. These are usually seen on the second or third day after the event (2.1).

d) F Signs of fat embolism include: pyrexia, cyanosis, pallor and dyspnoea (2.1).

e) T Fat emboli are sometimes seen in the retinal vessels on ophthalmoscopy and there may be petechial haemorrhages of the conjunctivae (2.1).

3a) T The action of non-depolarising muscle relaxants is potentiated by halothane. Halothane also potentiates the ganglion-blocking effects of tubocurarine which may produce hypotension (3.1).

b) F Soon after induction of anaesthesia with halothane there is a rise in skin temperature of up to 4°C and a fall in oesophageal temperature of up to 1°C. These changes are thought to be due to redistribution of blood flow (3.1).

c) T As halothane anaesthesia deepens there is a progressive reduction in renal blood flow and glomerular filtration rate. Urinary flow decreases and antidiuretic hormone release is stimulated (3.1).

d) T Enzymatic metabolism of halothane produces the following products which can be found in the plasma and urine: bromide, chloride, trifluoracetylethanolamide, chlorobromodifluoroethylene and trifluoroacetic acid (3.1).

e) T Trifluoroacetic acid is the main oxidative metabolite of halothane and is relatively non-toxic. It may take up to 3 weeks to completely clear halothane metabolites from the body (3.1).

4 Angina may be a symptom of:
a) aortic stenosis
b) anaemia
c) pericarditis
d) myxoedema
e) paroxysmal supraventricular tachycardia

5 Vasoconstriction is caused by:
a) phenoxybenzamine
b) angiotensin II
c) adenosine
d) angiotensin I
e) hypocarbia

6 Diazepam:
a) is water soluble
b) is less potent in the elderly
c) has a high therapeutic index
d) has more than one active metabolite
e) is an anticonvulsant

References

4.1	Souhami	p 383
4.2	Souhami	p 430
4.3	Souhami	p 400
4.4	Souhami	p 695
4.5	Souhami	p 366
5.1	Rang	p 200
5.2	Dundee	p 429
5.3	Dundee	p 397
5.4	Synopsis	p 79
6.1	Vickers	p 88–95

4a) T An increase in left ventricular work and thickening of the ventricular wall causes subendocardial ischaemia leading to angina. Angina can occur without pre-existing coronary atheroma (4.1).

b) T In anaemia the cardiac output increases to supply the oxygen requirements of the body and the heart is perfused with anaemic blood. This combination can result in continuous angina and heart failure (4.2).

c) F Acute pericarditis may cause severe chest pain which is exacerbated by movement, deep respiration and coughing. It can often be relieved by sitting forward and by non-steroidal anti-inflammatory drugs. These features can provide a clue to the diagnosis (4.3).

d) T Angina is an important sign in myxoedema as treatment can precipitate a myocardial infarct (4.4).

e) T Patients may complain of palpitations, breathlessness, dizziness, fatigue or chest pain (4.5).

5a) F Phenoxybenzamine causes a fall in arterial pressure due to vasodilation as alpha receptor-mediated vasoconstriction is blocked (5.1).

b) T Angiotensin II is the most powerful vasoconstrictor known. It is an active component of the renin-angiotensin system (5.2).

c) F Adenosine and adenosine triphosphate reduce systemic vascular resistance and can be used for the induction of hypotension (5.3).

d) F Angiotensin I is the inactive precursor of angiotensin II (5.2).

e) T Hypocarbia (hypocapnia) causes vasoconstriction (5.4).

6a) F Diazepam is insoluble in water. In its usual preparation diazepam is dissolved in an aqueous vehicle of organic solvents (propylene glycol, ethyl alcohol and sodium benzoate in benzoic acid) or a lipid vehicle (6.1).

b) F Sensitivity to the effects of benzodiazepines is increased in the elderly and in debilitated patients. The requirements are about half the usual dose and when given intravenously the injection should be no faster than 10 mg/min (6.1).

c) T The therapeutic index is the ratio of effective to lethal dose. Benzodiazepines have a high therapeutic index as even very large doses rarely result in serious side effects or death (6.1).

d) T Active metabolites are: desmethyldiazepam (with a half-life of 36–200 h) and oxazepam (with a half-life of 5–20 h). The half-life of diazepam is 20–50 h (6.1).

e) T Diazepam is the drug of first choice in all types of convulsions (6.1).

7 In Bier's technique (IVRA):
   a) 30 ml of 1.5% prilocaine is a suitable dose of local anaesthetic
   b) systemic effects of the local anaesthetic may be seen in the presence of a functioning cuff
   c) prilocaine is an unsuitable agent
   d) it is not necessary to starve the patient
   e) the cuff can be deflated after 10 minutes

8 The femoral nerve:
   a) is included in the '3 in 1' block
   b) gives off a branch to the skin of the scrotum
   c) lies medial to the femoral vein
   d) lies within the femoral sheath
   e) when blocked provides suitable anaesthesia for reduction of a fractured neck of femur

9 Passive hyperventilation leads to:
   a) metabolic acidosis
   b) reduction in serum calcium
   c) analgesia
   d) reduction in the potency of tubocurarine
   e) depletion of extracellular potassium

References	
7.1 Aitkenhead	p 464–465
7.2 Synopsis	p 648–650
8.1 Wildsmith	p 158–161
8.2 Gray's	p 1143
8.3 Gray's	p 1432
9.1 Synopsis	p 39–40

7a) F The maximum dose of prilocaine is 3–4 mg/kg, so assuming a standard weight of 70 kg the maximum volume of 1.5% prilocaine would be 14 ml. The recommended dose is 40 ml of 0.5% prilocaine (7.1).

b) T Rapid injection can result in the cuff pressure being exceeded and local anaesthetic solution entering the systemic circulation (7.1). Interosseous leakage may also occur (7.2).

c) F Prilocaine is the recommended agent (7.1). Bupivacaine should not be used because of its cardiotoxicity (7.2).

d) F The patient should be starved and intravenous access should be available in the opposite limb because systemic toxic effects of local anaesthetic will need treatment if they occur (7.1).

e) F The cuff should not be deflated before 20 min after injection of local anaesthetic. Cyclical inflation and deflation has been recommended (7.1).

8a) T The so called '3 in 1' block includes the femoral nerve, lateral cutaneous nerve of thigh and obturator nerve (8.1).

b) F The distribution of the branches of the femoral nerve do not include a branch to the scrotum (8.2). It is beyond the scope of this book to describe the details of the femoral nerve or the innervation of the scrotum (8.3).

c) F The femoral nerve lies behind and lateral to the sheath surrounding the femoral artery and vein (8.1).

d) F The sheath surrounds the vessels and excludes the nerve (8.1).

e) F Femoral nerve block is suitable for operations on the shaft of the femur distal to the upper third. The hip joint is supplied by a branch of the obturator nerve (8.1).

9a) F When the work of ventilation is at the expense of an external source ventilation is passive and there is no increase in carbon dioxide production. In active ventilation the respiratory effort increases muscle metabolism resulting in increased carbon dioxide production (9.1).
Moderate hyperventilation does not cause a 'significant' increase in metabolic acidosis or tissue hypoxia (9.1).

b) F There is a slight increase in total plasma calcium and a fall in ionized calcium (9.1).

c) T The threshold to pain may be increased threefold in volunteers and there is a reduction in requirements for analgesic agents (9.1).

d) F The potency of tubocurarine is increased and there is a reduction in dose requirements (9.1).

e) T Extracellular potassium is depleted. A small fall in plasma potassium may be seen (9.1).

10 Signs of adequate reversal of neuromuscular blockade include:
a) sustained head lift for 5 s
b) good tidal volume
c) normal arterial carbon dioxide
d) adequate minute volume
e) defence of airway on obstruction

11 Pulmonary oedema is associated with:
a) nitric oxide
b) atrial myxoma
c) air embolism
d) mitral stenosis
e) cardiomyopathy

12 Entonox:
a) can cause bone marrow depression
b) is stored as a liquid at 140 bar
c) separates into nitrous oxide and oxygen at 0°C
d) is licensed by the UKCC for unsupervised use by midwives
e) can be supplied by pipeline

References

10.1 Aitkenhead   p 427–428

11.1 Synopsis   p 134
11.2 Mason   p 243–251

12.1 Synopsis   p 137–138
12.2 Aitkenhead   p 272

10a) T Unlike the subjective grip strength and 'adequate cough', the ability of the patient to sustain a head lift for at least 5 s is an objective test of recovery from neuromuscular blockade (10.1).

b) F Measurement of an adequate tidal volume or minute volume in an unconscious patient is only a guide that recovery is occurring. The muscle power in partially paralysed patients may be sufficient for these parameters to approach normal (10.1).

c) F Reversal may be incomplete despite normal carbon dioxide tension (10.1).

d) F Adequate minute volume may only be a guide to impending recovery (10.1).

e) T The ability to produce a negative airway pressure of −20 cmH$_2$O against an obstructed airway constitutes a good test of recovery from neuromuscular blockade. (10.1).

11a) T The higher oxides of nitrogen, including nitric oxide and nitrogen dioxide, can occur as impurities of nitrous oxide. Such poisoning is very rare (two cases were described by Clutton-Brock in 1967). It appears in examinations more frequently (11.1).

b) T If there is left atrial outflow obstruction caused by an atrial myxoma or mitral valve stenosis the left atrial pressure will be high. The high pulmonary capillary pressure that results causes an increase in lung water thus producing pulmonary oedema (11.2).

c) T The mechanism for non-cardiogenic pulmonary oedema caused by air embolism has not been fully elucidated (11.2).

d) T Mitral valve stenosis results in high pulmonary capillary pressures as described in (b) (11.2).

e) T Cardiomyopathy leads to a reduction in left ventricular function and an increased afterload. Pulmonary capillary pressure will rise and pulmonary oedema will occur (11.2).

12a) T Bone marrow aplasia and fatal agranulocytosis have resulted from 'prolonged' exposure to nitrous oxide (12.1). As Entonox is a 50% mixture of nitrous oxide and oxygen it would be safe to assume that bone marrow depression is a side effect!

b) F Entonox is the BOC trade name for nitrous oxide 50% and oxygen 50%. It is stored in cylinders as a gas at a pressure of 137 bar at 15°C (12.2). The ability of nitrous oxide to remain in the gaseous phase when mixed with oxygen at pressures that would usually liquefy it is called the Poynting effect (12.1).

c) F Nitrous oxide starts to liquefy at −7°C. Use of a cylinder below this temperature will result in initial high oxygen concentrations followed by a hypoxic mixture (12.1).

d) T The United Kingdom Central Council (UKCC) permit its use by midwives on their own responsibility (12.1).

e) T Entonox can be supplied in cylinders or by pipeline (12.1).

13 Digoxin is suitable treatment in:
  a) hypertrophic cardiomyopathy
  b) supraventricular tachycardia
  c) cardiac amyloid
  d) first degree heart block
  e) cardiac tamponade

14 DC cardioversion is a recognised treatment for:
  a) ventricular fibrillation
  b) frequent ventricular ectopics
  c) conduction defects
  d) atrial fibrillation
  e) asystole

15 Drugs used in the treatment of paroxysmal supraventricular tachycardia include:
  a) verapamil
  b) nifedipine
  c) mexilitine
  d) lignocaine
  e) propranolol

References

| 13.1 Dundee | p 362 |
| 13.2 BNF | s 2.1.1 |

14.1 Davidson's	p 279
14.2 Davidson's	p 271
14.3 Davidson's	p 277–279
14.4 Davidson's	p 272–273
14.5 BMJ (1989) 299	p 446–8

| 15.1 Davidson's | p 274 |
| 15.2 BNF | s 2.6.2 |

13a) F Hypertrophic cardiomyopathy is a contraindication to therapy with digoxin due to an increase in outflow obstruction (13.1).

b) T The indications for the use of digoxin are heart failure and supraventricular arrhythmias (especially atrial fibrillation) (13.2).

c) F Digoxin reduces the electrical conductivity of the Purkinje system and thus will aggravate 2 to 1 heart block. Digoxin can cause atrioventricular block (13.2).

d) F Digoxin is contraindicated in cases of cardiac amyloid when arrhythmias may be precipitated (13.2).

e) F Although digoxin improves myocardial contractility, it will not be effective against the physical effects of tamponade (13.2).

14a) T Ventricular fibrillation is an emergency and the sooner the shock is applied the more likely it is to be successful (14.1).

b) F An underlying cause (such as escape beats during bradycardia) should be sought. If frequent ectopic beats without a cause are annoying the patient then beta blockade, disopyramide or mexiletine therapy may suppress them (14.2).

c) F There are many types of conduction defect none of which is treatable by cardioversion (14.3).

d) T Atrial fibrillation, atrial flutter and supraventricular tachycardia can be treated by DC (direct current) cardioversion (14.1).

e) F Asystole may respond to adrenaline or atropine. Temporary pacing may be successful. When drugs are given during a cardiac arrest, sufficient cardiac massage must be performed to ensure that the drugs have reached the cardiac conducting tissue (14.4). Resuscitation council (UK) recommendations infer that if there is doubt about the diagnosis then DC cardioversion should be used. If the true diagnosis is asystole then cardioversion is inappropriate (14.5).

15a) T Verapamil is used in the treatment of supraventricular tachycardia (SVT) and for the control of atrial fibrillation (AF). It is a class IV drug in the Vaughan-Williams classification (15.1).

b) F Nifedipine lacks antiarrhythmic activity and its calcium channel blocking activity is more pronounced in vessels than myocardium (15.2).

c) F Mexilitine is a class I drug which is useful in the treatment and prevention of ventricular tachyarrhythmias (15.1).

d) F Lignocaine is a class I drug used in the treatment and short-term prevention of ventricular tachycardia and fibrillation (15.1).

e) T Propranolol is a class II drug used in treatment and prevention of SVT and AF which can also be used in the prevention of ventricular ectopics and exercise-induced ventricular tachycardia (15.1).

16 **Prolonged high-dose glucocorticoid administration leads to:**
   a) muscle weakness
   b) water retention
   c) hypertension
   d) potassium depletion
   e) sodium retention

17 **Measures to decrease the incidence of suxamethonium pains include:**
   a) a small dose of suxamethonium pre-induction
   b) a small dose of non-depolarising muscle relaxant pre-induction
   c) dantrolene two hours pre-operatively
   d) concurrent intravenous fentanyl
   e) exercise prior to induction

18 **A hereditary enzyme abnormality may lead to altered metabolism of:**
   a) propofol
   b) aminophylline
   c) thiopentone
   d) suxamethonium
   e) atracurium

References	
16.1 Rang	p 517–519
16.2 Mason	p 61
17.1 Synopsis	p 209–210
18.1 Dundee	p 164–165
18.2 Dundee	p 592
18.3 Synopsis	p 394
18.4 Synopsis	p 206–208
18.5 Dundee	p 308

16a) T Prolonged glucocorticoid administration results in the clinical picture of Cushing's syndrome. Proximal muscle wasting and weakness occurs (16.1).

b) T The biochemical abnormalities of Cushing's syndrome include sodium and water retention, hypokalaemic alkalosis, hyperglycaemia and lack of diurnal variation in plasma cortisol (16.2).

c) T Hypertension can be a restricting factor in the use of steroids. Heart failure may also occur (16.1).

d) T Hypokalaemia may also lead to alkalosis (16.2).

e) T Sodium and water retention are seen (16.2).

17a) T 10 mg of suxamethonium followed by injection of the rest of the dose 1 min later reduces fasciculations and may reduce myalgia (17.1).

b) T Pre-curarization is the intravenous injection of a small dose of non-depolarising muscle relaxant 3 min before the suxamethonium (for example tubocurarine 3–5 mg or gallamine 5–20 mg) (17.1).

c) T A single oral dose of dantrolene (100–150 mg) at least 2 h pre-operatively reduces the incidence of muscle pains (17.1).

d) F All methods of reduction of pain involve drugs given before suxamethonium. Many drugs have been tried, recognised ones are cited in the reference (17.1).

e) F Pain is less frequent in those that are muscularly 'fit' than in the 'unfit' and pre-suxamethonium exercise is not a factor (17.1).

18a) F Propofol is metabolised to the glucuronide in the liver. The glucuronide is excreted in the urine (18.1).

b) F Methylxanthines are metabolised mainly by the liver. Plasma levels are measured because of the low therapeutic index (18.2).

c) F Beware. Thiopentone is metabolised in the liver. Porphyria is an hereditary enzyme abnormality in which thiopentone should not be used (18.3). There is no direct link between altered thiopentone metabolism and inheritance.

d) T Abnormal plasma cholinesterase (inherited) results in a reduction of the rate of hydrolysis of suxamethonium to succinyl monocholine and thence to choline and succinic acid (18.4).

e) T Ester hydrolysis is the main metabolic pathway so, in theory, atracurium can suffer the same problems as suxamethonium if the plasma cholinesterase is abnormal. In clinical practice, Hofmann degradation provides a 'safety net' (18.5).

19 Suxamethonium may cause:
a) bradycardia
b) histamine release
c) raised intraocular pressure
d) salivation
e) muscle pains

20 Airways resistance:
a) is constant
b) is decreased by propranolol
c) is increased by noradrenaline
d) is increased by parasympathetic stimulation
e) is mainly due to small airways

21 Atropine may cause:
a) vasodilation
b) diarrhoea
c) mydriasis
d) cycloplegia
e) hyperpyrexia

References		
19.1 Synopsis	p 204–210
20.1 Aitkenhead	p 29
20.2 Synopsis	p 308–309
20.3 Dundee	p 354
20.4 Guyton	p 672
20.5 West	p 105
21.1 Dundee	p 320–323
21.2 BNF	s 11.5

19a) T Bradycardia and cardiac arrest may occur on the first injection or, more commonly, on repeated administration (19.1).
  b) T Histamine release can occur without previous exposure, resulting in bronchospasm, hypotension, circulatory collapse and oedema (19.1).
  c) T Intraocular pressure will rise by 7 mmHg due to tonic contraction of the extraocular muscles. The pressure returns to normal in about 10 min due to absorption of aqueous humour (19.1).
  d) T Salivation and increased gastric secretion are muscarinic effects (19.1).
  e) T Muscle pains are more frequent in women, the middle-aged and the 'unfit' (19.1).

20a) F Resistance to airflow varies with tracheobronchial anatomy and type of gas flow. Gas flow may be laminar, transitional or turbulent (20.1).
  b) F Propranolol blocks sympathetically mediated bronchial dilatation and may cause severe bronchospasm with an increase in airway resistance (20.2).
  c) F Noradrenaline has no significant action at $beta_2$ receptors and so there will be no change in airway resistance (20.3).
  d) T Bronchi constrict with parasympathetic stimulation, thus airway resistance will rise (20.4).
  e) F Less than 20% of the total airway resistance can be attributed to airways smaller than 2 mm in diameter (20.5).

21a) T Vasodilation of cutaneous vessels is a direct effect that is unrelated to the muscarinic actions which will occur with large doses (21.1).
  b) F Atropine reduces the frequency and amplitude of peristalsis of all segments of the gastrointestinal tract (21.1).
  c) T Atropine has a mydriatic action secondary to the blockade of the responses of the sphincter muscle of the iris to acetylcholine, leaving the radial fibres unopposed (21.1).
  d) T Antimuscarinic drugs paralyse the ciliary muscle (21.2). It is important to differentiate between terms. Mydriasis means pupillary dilation; cycloplegia means ciliary muscle paralysis.
  e) T Atropine does not raise the temperature of normothermic volunteers. Suppression of sweating in high environmental temperatures and a possible central effect with very large doses may cause a rise in temperature but these are abnormal circumstances (21.1).

22 Atracurium:

a) is degraded by ester hydrolysis
b) is metabolised to laudanosine
c) in high doses acts faster than suxamethonium
d) is potentiated by alkalosis
e) is potentiated by hypothermia

23 Headache following spinal anaesthesia:

a) usually lasts longer than 24 h
b) is more likely if a 22 G needle is used rather than 26 G
c) is due to raised CSF pressure
d) is associated with VIth nerve palsy
e) can be treated with an epidural blood patch

24 Dopamine:

a) is a neurotransmitter
b) is formed from L-dopa as a precursor
c) crosses the blood–brain barrier
d) can be taken orally
e) decreases renal blood flow below a dose of 5 µg/kg.min^{-1}

References

22.1 Vickers		p 263–265
23.1 Synopsis		p 712–713
24.1 Vickers		p 224
24.2 Rang		p 699
24.3 Dundee		p 352

22a) T Atracurium is broken down by both Hofmann elimination and ester hydrolysis (22.1).

b) T Principal end products of metabolism are laudanosine and an acrylate ester (22.1).

c) F Although the onset of action is relatively short, there is a delay of 1.5–2 min before intubation conditions are ideal. This is slower than suxamethonium (22.1).

d) F Within a physiological pH range, changes of pH have 'little' effect (22.1).

e) T Doses should be reduced by approximately one third for a body temperature of 25°C. (22.1).

23a) T The headache may last days, weeks or months but usually about 1–2 weeks (23.1).

b) T The incidence of headache increases with increasing size of needle; dural puncture with a Tuohy needle will result in a headache in 75% of patients, 22 G needle 20% and 25 G needle 3.5% (23.1).

c) T There are at least two theories of causation: low CSF pressure and high CSF pressure (23.1). A reduction in CSF pressure occurs as a result of a CSF leak and an increase in CSF pressure occurs as a result of meningeal irritation. The former theory is most widely held.

d) T VIth nerve palsy can occur resulting in paralysis of the external rectus and diplopia. Paralysis of every cranial nerve except the Ist, IXth and Xth have been reported (23.1).

e) T A 92% success rate has been claimed for epidural blood patches at the correct level (23.1). It is believed that a blood patch stops CSF leakage and increases CSF pressure. It is necessary to subscribe to the low CSF pressure causation theory before performing a blood patch.

24a) T Dopamine is a central and peripheral neurotransmitter, acting on both D_1 and D_2 receptors (24.1).

b) T L-Dopa, the L isomer of dopa or levodopa is used in the treatment of Parkinson's disease. L-Dopa is metabolised to dopamine both peripherally and centrally but crosses the blood-brain barrier whereas dopamine will not (24.2).

c) F Dopamine does not cross the blood-brain barrier. See (b) above (24.2).

d) F Dopamine is administered only by the intravenous route. The wall of the intestine contains monoamine oxidase which would inactivate dopamine (24.2).

e) F If dopamine is administered at a rate of 2–3 $\mu g/kg.min^{-1}$ renal and mesenteric vasodilation occurs. This effect may occur up to 5 $\mu g/kg.min^{-1}$. Renal blood flow increases as does urine flow (if the circulating volume has been restored) (24.3).

25 In arterial cannulation:
  a) the right radial artery should be used in preference to the left
  b) a parallel sided cannula is preferable
  c) a 14 G or 16 G cannula is suitable
  d) Allen's test should be performed
  e) ischaemic necrosis is a sequel

26 Symptoms associated with epidural block to T10 are:
  a) slow heart rate
  b) vagal block
  c) motor paralysis
  d) prolonged analgesia
  e) Horner's syndrome

27 Latent heat of vaporisation:
  a) is lower at high temperatures
  b) is the heat required to change a liquid to a vapour
  c) is zero at the critical temperature
  d) SI units are joules kg^{-1}
  e) is responsible for the majority of heat loss from the respiratory tract

---

References

25.1 Aitkenhead		p 369–371
25.2 Synopsis		p 349
26.1 Aitkenhead		p 465–467
26.2 Synopsis		p 729
27.1 Parbrook		p 126–129
27.2 Parbrook		p 131–132

25a) F If possible, the non-dominant hand should be used. Assuming the majority of patients to be right handed then the left hand should be used (25.1).

b) T A Teflon, parallel sided cannula of small diameter and the use of Luer Lok connections are recommended (25.1).

c) F A 20 G or 22 G needle is recommended to minimise trauma (25.1).

d) T The patency of the ulnar artery is confirmed by Allen's test before the radial artery is punctured (25.2).

e) T Possible sequelae of long-term arterial cannulation include: arterial wall damage and thrombosis, embolisation, disconnection and haemorrhage, sepsis and tissue necrosis (25.1).

26a) T There is a reduction in heart rate when plain local anaesthetic solutions are used. Note, however, that the use of adrenaline-containing solutions results in maintenance of heart rate or a tachycardia (26.1).

b) F Denervation of the sympathetic outflow occurs. The vagal (parasympathetic) nerve supply remains intact, resulting in unopposed parasympathetic action on the gastrointestinal tract, so producing a constricted gut with increased peristaltic activity (26.1).

c) T Although differential blockade occurs, motor blockade will occur up to a level two segments caudal to the upper level of a sensory block (26.1).

d) T 60 h of analgesia has been reported after 18 ml of 0.5% bupivacaine plain (26.2).

e) T Recovery from Horner's syndrome may be delayed (26.2).

27a) T Specific latent heat is defined as the heat required to convert 1 kg of a substance from one phase to another at a given temperature. The higher the temperature the less latent heat is needed to vaporize a substance (27.1).

b) T Do not look for a deeper meaning. This is a description of latent heat of vaporisation (27.1).

c) T At its critical temperature a substance changes spontaneously from liquid to vapour without the supply of any external energy (27.1).

d) T The Systeme International (SI) units are $J.kg^{-1}$ or Joules/kg (27.1).

e) T In a person breathing dry gases at 7 l. min^{-1} heat loss due to humidification is nearly 10 W, whereas heat loss due to heating of the gases is 2 W (27.2).

28 In myocardial contraction:
a) the mitral valve closes before the tricuspid valve
b) the pulmonary valve closes before the aortic valve
c) the A-V valve cusps are stationary during ventricular filling
d) atrial contraction has a more significant effect on ventricular filling at increased heart rates
e) contractility is decreased by sympathetic stimulation

29 Atrial fibrillation is associated with:
a) mitral stenosis
b) left auricular thrombus
c) multiple P waves on the ECG
d) thyrotoxicosis
e) ischaemic heart disease

30 The following occur during exercise:
a) increased body temperature
b) increased diastolic pressure
c) potassium loss
d) decreased stroke volume
e) increased renal blood flow

References	
28.1 Ganong	p 521–526
29.1 Davidson's	p 270–272
30.1 Ganong	p 585–588
30.2 Guyton	p 948–949

28a) F At the start of ventricular systole the mitral and tricuspid (atrioventricular) valves close at the same time (28.1).

b) F During expiration both valves close at the same time but during inspiration the aortic valve closes slightly before the pulmonary valve (28.1).

c) F The cusps of the A-V valves drift towards the closed positions during ventricular filling (28.1).

d) T Most ventricular filling occurs in diastole. As diastole is shorter in tachycardia the importance of atrial systole is emphasised (28.1).

e) F The effect of sympathetic stimulation is to increase myocardial contractility (28.1).

29a) T Many types of valvular pathology are associated with atrial fibrillation, particularly mitral disease (29.1).

b) T Left auricular thrombus may develop. This presents a risk of systemic embolisation (29.1).

c) F The ECG is marked by a <u>lack</u> of P waves (29.1).

d) T Thyrotoxicosis is associated with atrial fibrillation (29.1).

e) T Ischaemic heart disease is an association of atrial fibrillation (29.1).

30a) T Body temperature rises due to the inability of the heat dissipation mechanisms to cope with the increased metabolism (30.1).

b) F Diastolic pressure may remain unchanged or fall (30.1).

c) T Heavy exercise, especially in conditions of high ambient temperature results in marked potassium loss due mainly to the action of aldosterone (30.2).

d) F Stroke volume is increased (30.1).

e) F Renal blood flow falls during exercise (30.1).

31 **The following statements are true of soda lime:**
   a) 20% volume for volume of soda lime is sodium hydroxide
   b) 90% is calcium carbonate
   c) water is necessary for the reaction
   d) the reaction with carbon dioxide is exothermic
   e) soda lime fills half a Waters' canister

32 **During ERPOC (evacuation of retained products of conception) reduced uterine tone may be caused by:**
   a) fentanyl
   b) enflurane
   c) syntocinon
   d) nitrous oxide
   e) propofol

33 **Immediate treatment of anaphylaxis includes:**
   a) corticosteroid administration
   b) 0.5 mg adrenaline i.v.
   c) oxygen
   d) prochlorperazine i.m.
   e) aminophylline i.v.

References	
31.1 Aitkenhead	p 306–307
32.1 Aitkenhead	p 487
33.1 Mason	p 450–451

31a) F The major constituent of soda lime is calcium hydroxide (94%). There is 5% vol/vol sodium hydroxide in soda lime (31.1).

b) F Calcium carbonate is the end product of the reaction on absorption of carbon dioxide by soda lime (31.1).

c) T Water is required for efficient absorption. Some water is present in soda lime but water is also a product of the reaction and is present in the patient's expired gas (31.1).

d) T The reaction produces heat and is therefore exothermic. This property is cited as an advantage as it reduces patient heat loss by warming the gases (31.1).

e) F Unless the canister is packed tightly, when used horizontally, gas can pass above the soda lime so producing 'channelling' (31.1).

32a) F Fentanyl is frequently used in anaesthesia for ERPOC (32.1). Uterine relaxation does not result.

b) T Halothane, enflurane and isoflurane will all cause uterine relaxation and their use is not recommended for ERPOC when good uterine contraction is required (32.1).

c) F Syntocinon 5–10 units i.v. is used to produce uterine contraction. Beware of looking for deeper meanings in simple questions (32.1).

d) F Oxygen and nitrous oxide mixtures are regularly used for maintenance of anaesthesia during this procedure, without deleterious effect (32.1).

e) F Propofol is used for induction and sometimes in incremental i.v. boluses for maintenance during anaesthesia for ERPOC or termination of pregnancy (32.1). Uterine tone is largely unaffected.

33a) F The onset of action of corticosteroids at the cellular level may take several hours. Corticosteroids are recommended as second line treatment when resolution is slow and hypotension persists (33.1).

b) T Adrenaline is the drug of first choice and should be given early. Intravenous doses of 0.1–0.5 mg (0.1–0.5 ml of 1:1000 solution) or 5 µg/kg are quoted (33.1).

c) T Following cessation of administration of the suspected drug, the next action is to maintain the airway and give 100% oxygen (33.1).

d) F Prochlorperazine plays no part in the treatment of anaphylaxis. In addition, it is inappropriate to use the intramuscular route of drug administration for shocked patients because the absorption is unreliable or non-existent (33.1).

e) F Aminophylline is a drug of second line treatment which is indicated if bronchospasm persists (33.1).

34 Anaphylactoid reactions:
a) are more common with methohexitone than thiopentone
b) are more common in females
c) always involve C3 consumption
d) are invariably accompanied by bronchospasm
e) are common with local anaesthetic agents

35 In haemophilia:
a) a haemorrhagic rash is present
b) whole blood clotting time is altered
c) partial thromboplastin time is altered
d) bleeding time is prolonged
e) haemarthroses may be seen

36 Nitrous oxide:
a) is stored as a liquid at room temperature
b) is manufactured by heating ammonium nitrate
c) may be contaminated by nitric oxide
d) contaminants can be tested for by using starch iodide paper
e) in continuous use the pressure in a cylinder only falls when nearly empty

References

34.1 Mason   p 446–449

35.1 Mason   p 124

36.1 Aitkenhead   p 168–169
36.2 Dundee   p 127
36.3 Synopsis   p 132–135

34a) **F** Thiopentone causes more reactions than methohexitone, whereas etomidate is considered to be 'immunologically safe' (34.1).
 b) **T** 70% of serious cases occurred in women in one French study (34.1).
 c) **F** Non-immune anaphylactoid responses are common. These do not involve consumption of complement C3 and C4, as chemical mediators are released as a result of a direct or an indirect effect on mast cells and basophils without complement involvement (34.1).
 d) **F** Approximately 40% of anaphylactoid reactions involve bronchospasm. Note, however, it can be serious and result in death (34.1).
 e) **F** The incidence of true allergy is very low although it is often difficult to differentiate between toxicity and anaphylactoid response (34.1).

35a) **F** In mild haemophiliac states bleeding is usually a result of trauma. In severe haemophilia the majority of spontaneous bleeding episodes principally affect joints and muscles (35.1).
 b) **F** Whole blood clotting time is usually normal except in the most severe cases of haemophilia (35.1).
 c) **T** The inherited defect results in an abnormality of the intrinsic pathway with a prolongation of the partial thromboplastin time (PTT) (35.1).
 d) **F** The bleeding time is normal (35.1).
 e) **T** Spontaneous bleeding mainly affects the joints and muscles. Recurrent haemarthroses may lead to ankylosis and permanent joint deformities (35.1).

36a) **T** When compressed to the storage pressure of 50 bar (5000 kPa) nitrous oxide is in a liquid form (36.1).
 b) **T** Commercial manufacture involves heating ammonium nitrate to a temperature of 245–270°C (36.1).
 c) **T** Impurities produced during the manufacturing process include ammonia, nitric acid, nitrogen, nitric oxide and nitrogen dioxide (36.1). Impurities are removed by cooling the gas and passing it through water, caustic permanganate and acid scrubbers (36.2).
 d) **T** Moistened starch iodide paper exposed for 10 min to the suspect gas mixed with 25% oxygen will turn blue if the contamination is over 300 parts per million (assuming there is some starch iodide paper to hand) (36.3).
 e) **F** Latent heat is required for vaporisation; thus as gas is released the cylinder cools, and pressure within falls. With rapid flows (10 l/min) there is a linear fall in pressure. However, with low flows (2 l/min) there is a small but progressive decrease (36.3).

37 Bupivacaine:
a) is a local anaesthetic of the amide group
b) is metabolised by plasma cholinesterase
c) can cause methaemoglobinaemia
d) has a recommended maximum dose of 2 mg/kg
e) can be used for post-operative pain relief

38 Diamorphine:
a) is rapidly hydrolysed to morphine
b) is more lipid soluble than morphine
c) causes nausea and vomiting by acting on the chemoreceptor trigger zone
d) causes myocardial depression
e) is stable in solution

39 Mendelson's syndrome is associated with:
a) pulmonary oedema
b) urticarial rash
c) bronchospasm
d) cyanosis
e) methaemoglobinaemia

References	
37.1 Dundee	p 283–293
37.2 Aitkenhead	p 455
38.1 Dundee	p 208–214
39.1 Synopsis	p 523–525
39.2 Synopsis	p 432

37a) T Bupivacaine is a member of the amide group of local anaesthetic agents (37.1).
  b) F The ester group are metabolised by plasma cholinesterase. The amide type agents are metabolised in the liver with small amounts being excreted via the kidneys (37.1).
  c) F It is prilocaine that is well known as a cause of methaemoglobinaemia (37.1).
  d) T The recommended maximum dose is 2 mg/kg over a 4-hour period (37.1).
  e) T A relatively long duration of action makes bupivacaine suitable for post-operative pain relief (37.3).

38a) F Diamorphine is rapidly metabolised in the plasma and tissues to monoacetylmorphine (MAM) and then to morphine by deacetylation, not by hydrolysis (38.1).
  b) T Diamorphine and monoacetylmorphine are both more lipid soluble than morphine. They may act as 'carriers' of morphine into the central nervous system (38.1).
  c) T Vomiting occurs as a result of stimulation of the chemoreceptor trigger zone, although stimulation of the vestibular nerve may be responsible for some of the nausea (38.1).
  d) F The hypotension associated with diamorphine and morphine is due to vasodilatation. There is little effect on the myocardium (38.1).
  e) F When in solution, diamorphine rapidly undergoes deacetylation (38.1).

39a) T Mendelson described the acid aspiration syndrome of late pregnancy (39.1). The respiratory and vascular epithelia are damaged with the result that fluid leaks into the alveoli and interstitial spaces. The increased water in the lungs results in pulmonary oedema (39.1).
  b) F The signs and symptoms are cyanosis, dyspnoea, tachycardia, bronchospasm, pulmonary oedema and acute respiratory failure (39.2).
  c) T Bronchospasm may not occur for some hours (39.1).
  d) T The cyanosis is unrelieved by oxygen therapy (39.1).
  e) F Methaemoglobinaemia is not a feature of acid aspiration syndrome (39.2).

40 The following may be associated with pyloric stenosis:
a) hypokalaemia
b) low plasma chloride
c) high plasma urea
d) low plasma bicarbonate
e) high haematocrit

41 The following are reduced in the elderly patient:
a) functional residual capacity
b) arterial oxygen tension
c) alveolar oxygen tension
d) forced expiratory volume
e) MAC of halothane

42 The following local anaesthetic agents cause significant vasoconstriction:
a) cocaine
b) amethocaine
c) bupivacaine
d) lignocaine
e) prilocaine

References		
40.1 Zilva	p 97–98	
41.1 Davenport	p 22–23	
41.2 Davenport	p 40–41	
41.3 Davenport	p 50	
42.1 Dundee	p 291–293	
42.2 Wildsmith	p 23–35	

40a) T The hypokalaemia which may be seen is due to vomiting with consequent potassium loss. This is aggravated by the alkalosis which is secondary to direct loss of hydrogen ions (40.1).

b) T Hypochloraemic alkalosis is a classic biochemical feature of pyloric stenosis. Chloride loss from the lumen of the stomach is direct and may be substantial (40.1).

c) T Uraemia is often present but usually mild. It is inevitably due to volume depletion (40.1).

d) F The prevailing situation is one of alkalosis. The plasma bicarbonate will thus be elevated. The elevation appears more marked in the usual situation of dehydration (40.1).

e) T For the reasons described above (40.1).

41a) F Although inspiratory and expiratory reserve volumes decrease (and therefore vital capacity also), FRC is thought to be increased in the elderly (41.1).

b) T Arterial oxygen tension falls with age. Lung damage accrued over a period of years will lead to a fall in both P_{AO_2} and P_{aO_2} (41.1).

c) T See (b) above (41.2).

d) T Forced expiratory volume and vital capacity are reduced (41.2).

e) T The MAC value for all the volatile anaesthetic agents is reduced in the elderly population (41.3).

42a) T Cocaine is a powerful vasoconstrictor. This effect is used prior to ENT surgery, on the nose for example (42.1).

b) F The majority of the local anaesthetic agents are vasodilators, the two major exceptions being cocaine and prilocaine (42.2).

c) F Bupivacaine is a vasodilator (42.2).

d) F Lignocaine has a significant vasodilating action (42.2).

e) F Prilocaine is unusual among the local anaesthetic agents in being neither a vasoconstrictor nor a vasodilator (42.2).

43 Tracheostomy:
a) is indicated in airway obstruction
b) increases anatomical dead space
c) may cause tracheal stenosis
d) removes the need for humidified gases
e) may become infected

44 The following factors increase the risk of DVT:
a) obesity
b) polycythaemia
c) malignancy
d) heparin
e) oral contraceptive medication

45 Blood filters:
a) have a pore size of 100 microns
b) may be screen or depth types
c) may damage red cells
d) become less efficient with each unit passed
e) remove microaggregates

References	
43.1 Synopsis	p 807–810
44.1 Synopsis	p 266–268
45.1 Ward	p 297–298

43a) T Indications for tracheostomy include: upper airway obstruction, prevention of aspiration and need for tracheobronchial toilet (43.1).
b) F After tracheostomy, anatomical dead space is reduced by approximately 30–50% in value (43.1).
c) T One of the later complications of tracheostomy is the development of tracheal stenosis. This often follows on from the development of tracheal ulceration secondary to direct irritation from tubes (43.1).
d) F Since the nasal passages and oropharynx have been by-passed, the need for humidification of administered gases is greater than previously (43.1).
e) T As with any surgical procedure, infection is a constant risk (43.1).

44a) T Obesity is a well known risk factor for the development of DVT (44.1).
b) T Polycythaemia increases the risk of DVT (44.1). In polycythaemia rubra vera thrombotic incidents are very common.
c) T Malignant disease increases the likelihood of the development of DVT (44.1).
d) F Heparin is used as a prophylactic drug to reduce the incidence of DVT after surgery. Commonly subcutaneous doses are employed in the pre- and early post-operative periods (44.1).
e) T Contraceptive medication carries an increased risk of DVT development. This may be defrayed by the use of heparin pre-operatively (44.1).

45a) F The usual pore size of blood filters lies between 20 and 40 microns (45.1).
b) T There are two main types of filter. Screen types have a pleated sheet of polyester acting as a sieve. Depth filters are packed fibres in a container. The two types may be met as a single unit (45.1).
c) T All available blood filters carry the risk of red cell damage. This is more marked when they are combined with pressure infusing devices to increase flow (45.1).
d) F Take care. As screen filters clog the effective pore size is reduced and efficiency increases. This obviously only holds true up to a certain point! Depth filters become less efficient with each successive unit transfused (45.1).
e) T Removal of particles is the main reason for using a blood filter. The majority of microaggregates are not removed by the standard giving set filter (45.1).

46 Renal blood flow:
a) is one fifth of cardiac output at rest
b) is decreased by IPPV
c) is evenly distributed throughout the kidney
d) is constant between arterial pressures of 75–160 mmHg
e) decreases with halothane

47 The following are physiological responses to plasma loss:
a) decreased baroreceptor discharge
b) arteriolar constriction
c) venous constriction
d) increased formation of angiotensin II
e) increased formation of antidiuretic hormone

48 The oxygen-haemoglobin dissociation curve moves to the right:
a) with an increase in temperature
b) when 2,3-DPG levels increase
c) when carbon dioxide concentration increases
d) with an increase in hydrogen ion concentration
e) on exercise

References	
46.1 Guyton	p 288–293
46.2 Nunn	p 418–419
46.3 Synopsis	p 138–141
47.1 Guyton	p 264–268
47.2 Guyton	p 198
48.1 Guyton	p 438

46a) T In a 70 kg man the normal blood flow through both kidneys is about 1200 ml/min. The cardiac output is about 5600 ml/min. The portion of total cardiac output that passes through the kidneys is called the renal fraction. It is about 21% but may vary from 12% to 30% (46.1).

b) T In Intermittent Positive Pressure Ventilation (IPPV) arterial pressure is reduced and central venous pressure is raised. Therefore the pressure gradient between renal artery and vein is reduced, so reducing renal blood flow (46.2).

c) F Only 1–2% of total renal blood flow perfuses the vasa recta of the medulla. Blood flow is rapid in the cortex and slow in the medulla (46.1).

d) T Renal blood flow and glomerular filtration rate is little changed over the normal systolic blood pressure range of 75–160 mmHg (46.1).

e) T There is a progressive reduction in renal blood flow as halothane concentration rises (46.3%).

47a) T Shock as a result of plasma loss has the same characteristics as haemorrhagic shock but blood viscosity also increases (47.1). Blood pressure will fall and baroreceptor discharge decrease as pressure falls, until there is no discharge at all below 60 mmHg (47.2).

b) T Arterioles constrict in most parts of the body, which results in an increase in total peripheral resistance and a rise in blood pressure (47.1).

c) T There is constriction of the veins and the venous reservoirs so increasing venous return (47.1).

d) T Angiotensin constricts peripheral arteries and causes increased conservation of water and salt by the kidneys (47.1).

e) T Antidiuretic hormone (vasopressin) constricts the peripheral arteries and veins and increases water retention by the kidneys (47.1).

48a) T It is important to be able to draw the curve and place on it the 'key' points. Drawing a rough diagram before answering this question may avoid confusion. An <u>increase</u> in any factor causes a shift to the right (48.1).

b) T 2,3-DPG (2,3-diphosphoglycerate) is a phosphate compound that increases in concentration during hypoxia lasting more than a few hours (48.1).

c) T The effect of carbon dioxide on the curve is called the Bohr effect (48.1).

d) T An increase in hydrogen ions, otherwise expressed as a decrease in pH, results in a shift to the right (48.1).

e) T Exercise results in an increase in temperature, carbon dioxide, hydrogen ions and phosphate ion release from the exercising muscle. The curve therefore moves to the right (48.1).

49 Enflurane:
   a) is an halogenated ether
   b) has a MAC value of 0.75
   c) is metabolised to fluoride ions
   d) has a boiling point of 50°C
   e) is irritant to the airway

50 Halothane:
   a) is an halogenated ether
   b) has a boiling point of 50°C
   c) delays cardiac conduction
   d) is metabolised to bromide ions
   e) is suitable for gaseous induction

51 Isoflurane:
   a) is a respiratory depressant
   b) is an halogenated ether
   c) has a MAC value of 0.76
   d) is metabolised less than halothane
   e) is a vasodilator

References	
49.1 Dundee	p 104–108
50.1 Dundee	p 113–119
51.1 Dundee	p 108–110

49a) T Enflurane is 2-chloro-1,2,2-trifluoroethyl-difluoromethyl ether (49.1).
b) F The MAC value for enflurane (in 100% oxygen) is 1.68% in adult patients (49.1).
c) T Fluorinated ethers such as enflurane are usually broken down in the liver to non-volatile metabolites, one of which is fluoride ions. Serum fluoride concentrations after enflurane anaesthesia are usually less than the nephrotoxic level of 50 μmol/l (49.1).
d) F The boiling point of enflurane at one atmosphere ambient pressure is 56°C (49.1).
e) F Enflurane is said to be non-irritant to the respiratory tract at clinically used concentrations (49.1). Regular clinical users of the vapour may wish to disagree with this statement.

50a) F Halothane is an halogenated hydrocarbon, not an ether, because it lacks an etheric bond (50.1).
b) T The boiling point of halothane at one atmosphere ambient pressure is 50.2°C (50.1).
c) T The effect of halothane on cardiac conducting tissue is to slow conduction. Ventricular automaticity is particularly depressed. The sensitising effect of halothane on the myocardium with resulting arrhythmias is well known (50.1).
d) T Bromide is produced by both reductive and oxidative pathways of metabolism. In contrast, only the reductive path yields significant amounts of fluoride (50.1).
e) T The non-irritant effect of halothane on the airway (50.1) makes it particularly useful for gaseous induction.

51a) T Isoflurane is depressant to respiration in a more profound manner than halothane, but less so than enflurane (51.1).
b) T Isoflurane is 1-chloro-2,2,2-trifluoroethyl difluoromethyl ether. It is a structural isomer of enflurane (51.1).
c) F The MAC value for isoflurane in 100% oxygen is 1.15% (51.1).
d) T The metabolism of isoflurane is minimal (51.1). In value it approximates to one tenth as much as halothane.
e) T The effect of isoflurane on peripheral resistance is to reduce it (51.1). Vasodilatation is seen in most vascular beds.

52 The following agents may cause methaemoglobinaemia:
a) prilocaine
b) sulphonamides
c) nitrites
d) phenacetin
e) ascorbic acid

53 Thiopentone sodium:
a) is an oxybarbiturate
b) dilates cerebral vessels
c) is acidic in solution
d) is used as a 5% solution
e) may cause hypotension

54 Alcuronium:
a) is a depolarising muscle relaxant
b) may cause hypotension
c) causes the release of histamine
d) is less potent than curare
e) may be reversed by edrophonium

References	
52.1 Synopsis	p 389
53.1 Synopsis	p 160–167
54.1 Dundee	p 304–305
54.2 Dundee	p 337

52a) T Methaemoglobinaemia is the presence of ferric haemoglobin, which is formed when the ferrous form of iron within the haem molecule becomes oxidised. The condition may be idiopathic or secondary to administered agents. In the list in this question the first four are agents which may cause methaemoglobinaemia but (e) is false. Vitamin C, ascorbic acid, is a treatment not a cause (52.1).

b) T See (a) above (52.1).

c) T See (a) above (52.1).

d) T See (a) above (52.1).

e) F An agent which may be used in the treatment of methaemoglobinaemia (52.1).

53a) F Thiopentone is a thiobarbiturate not an oxybarbiturate. The most commonly encountered oxybarbiturate in practice is methohexitone (53.1).

b) F The action of thiopentone on cerebral vasculature is constriction. This action is employed in the use of the agent to reduce intracranial pressure (53.1).

c) F To aid solubility thiopentone solution is severely alkaline. The pKa value of thiopentone (7.8) indicates that at plasma pH it will be less ionised and thus less water soluble (53.1).

d) F Although formerly this was the case, for many years thiopentone has been used as a 2.5% solution. This minimises the damage from accidental intra-arterial injection (53.1).

e) T Cardiac output is reduced and capacitance vessels are dilated. A combination of these events leads to systemic hypotension (53.1).

54a) F Alcuronium is a non-depolarising (competitive) muscle relaxant drug (54.1).

b) T Alcuronium causes hypotension in a dose-dependent manner (54.1). This is thought to be due to ganglion blockade in a similar fashion to curare.

c) T Although the effect is less than that seen after the administration of curare (54.1).

d) F Alcuronium is more potent than curare. Relative doses for intubation are: alcuronium 0.2 mg/kg, curare 0.4 mg/kg (54.1).

e) T In sufficiently high dose, edrophonium will reverse the effects of any of the non-depolarising relaxant drugs (54.2).

55 Surgical diathermy:
a) requires a large plate area
b) uses a sinusoidal waveform
c) requires the plate to be sited over an area with good blood supply
d) operates at frequencies below 400 kHz
e) always requires an earth

56 With respect to humidifiers:
a) ideal droplet size is one micron diameter
b) there is a risk of scalding
c) the Bernoulli effect is employed
d) water baths are more efficient than nebulisers
e) infection may be introduced

57 Nitrous oxide:
a) is manufactured by fractional distillation
b) has a boiling point of 89°C
c) may cause agranulocytosis
d) is eliminated by the lungs
e) has a critical temperature of 36.5°F

References	
55.1 Ward	p 334–337
56.1 Ward	p 242–247
57.1 Synopsis	p 132–137

55a) T The plate area should be as large as is practically possible. This will minimise the heating effect which tends to occur at the patient–plate interface (55.1).
  b) T A sinusoidal current is the normal for cutting diathermy. Coagulation usually employs a damped waveform version (55.1).
  c) T The reasoning being identical to that described above in (a). Placement under the buttocks is recommended but other sites may be employed when circumstances demand (55.1).
  d) F The frequencies at which surgical diathermy operates are not standardised. These vary, however, between 0.4–1.5 mHz (55.1).
  e) F Bipolar diathermy, in which the current passes from one forcep tip to another, is an earth-free system which is in contrast to the unipolar systems (55.1).

56a) F To achieve humidification of the trachea and bronchi requires droplets with a diameter of 1–10 microns. One-micron droplets tend to reach the alveoli without condensing out. This limits their usefulness (56.1).
  b) T Scalding is a constant risk and equipment is usually designed with complex thermostatic fail-safe devices to prevent it occurring (56.1).
  c) T The Bernoulli effect is seen as a pressure drop in a tube at its narrowest point. This effect is used in many humidifiers. For an example see reference (56.1).
  d) F The nebuliser is a very much more efficient humidifier than the water bath (56.1).
  e) T Infection is a constant risk. The humid and warm environment produced by the devices may encourage the growth of pathogens, *Pseudomonas* species for example (56.1).

57a) F The manufacturing process involves the heating of ammonium nitrate in a retort to 240°C (57.1).
  b) F Beware! The boiling point of nitrous oxide is <u>minus</u> 89 degrees Celsius (57.1).
  c) T Agranulocytosis is only a possibility in long-term usage. It may be a reflection of the interference of nitrous oxide with the metabolism of folate (57.1).
  d) T Nitrous oxide is eliminated unchanged through the lungs. This is the major route of excretion of the agent (57.1).
  e) F Another distractor. The critical temperature of nitrous oxide is 36.5 degrees <u>Celsius</u> (57.1).

58 Nasal intubation:
a) requires a larger diameter tube
b) should be performed through the right nostril
c) may cause bleeding
d) is suitable for ENT procedures
e) may aid IPPV

59 The following statements apply to day case anaesthesia:
a) ASA 3 patients are suitable
b) driving may be permitted within 24 h
c) starvation is not mandatory
d) intubation is acceptable
e) all cases should be seen by the anaesthetist before discharge

60 The lower oesophageal sphincter (LOS) pressure may be reduced by:
a) ethanol
b) morphine
c) suxamethonium
d) thiopentone
e) tricyclic antidepressant drugs

References	
58.1 Aitkenhead	p 358
59.1 Aitkenhead	p 519–526
60.1 Aitkenhead	p 530

58a) F Nasal intubation should be performed with a tube of internal diameter less than that for orotracheal intubation (58.1). A nasal tube will also need to be longer.

b) T It is said that the right nostril is preferential due to the left facing bevel on nasotracheal tubes (58.1).

c) T Haemorrhage may result from trauma to the turbinates, palate or even undiagnosed carcinoma within the nose. Occasionally the presence of unsuspected nasal polyps may cause severe bleeding.

d) T Improved surgical access makes nasal intubation very suitable for ENT surgery (58.1).

e) T Mainly because of the ease of fixation of nasal tubes which makes this route of intubation desirable for long-term intensive care patients requiring ventilation of their lungs (58.1).

59a) T Somewhat debatable. In general, most guidelines state ASA 1 and 2 categories as the minimum for day case surgery. Short procedures may, however, be suitable for some patients falling within ASA category 3 (59.1).

b) F Driving should be forbidden within 24 hours of the commencement of anaesthesia (59.1).

c) F The normal standards apply equally to day case anaesthesia. Starvation for six hours is recommended (59.1).

d) T The need for intubation should not be seen as an absolute contraindication (59.1). Long periods of intubation are not desirable.

e) T It is essential that the patient is seen and declared 'street fit' before discharge. Regrettably there is no good definition of this concept (59.1).

60a) T The lower oesophageal sphincter (LOS) is an area of higher intraluminal pressure found close to the cardia. It represents an effective barrier to regurgitation. Several drugs affect the tone of the LOS and ethanol reduces it (60.1).

b) T Opioids generally reduce the tone of the LOS (60.1).

c) F Suxamethonium was formerly thought to render regurgitation more likely due to the rise in gastric pressure which it induces. It is now clear that an accompanying rise in LOS pressure mitigates this effect (60.1).

d) T Thiopentone reduces the tone of the LOS (60.1).

e) T The tricyclic antidepressant agents reduce the tone of the LOS (60.1).

61 Pancuronium:
a) releases histamine
b) increases arterial pressure
c) is a monoquaternary compound
d) causes tachycardia
e) crosses the blood–brain barrier

62 Entonox:
a) demonstrates the Poynting effect
b) is stored at 100 atm
c) contains 60% nitrous oxide in air
d) is supplied in blue cylinders
e) has a boiling point of −80°C

63 Atropine:
a) crosses the blood–brain barrier
b) increases dead space
c) is a bronchoconstrictor
d) causes pyrexia
e) may cause bradycardia

References

61.1 Dundee	p 305–306
62.1 Ward	p 6
62.2 Dunnill	p 8
62.3 Synopsis	p 137–138
62.4 Ward	p 33
63.1 Dundee	p 318–323

61a) T Histamine release is quoted as 'minimal'. There is thus some uncertainty over the correct response. True is the author's choice (61.1). See question 294.

b) T Pancuronium causes an increase in arterial pressure which is likely to be due to a sympathetic stimulatory effect (61.1).

c) F Pancuronium is a bisquaternary, not monoquaternary, compound (61.1).

d) T The heart rate and arterial pressure both rise after a dose of pancuronium. See above (61.1).

e) F In common with all quaternary ammonium compounds, pancuronium does not cross the blood–brain barrier.

62a) T The Poynting effect is an effect whereby the critical temperature and critical pressure of one gas are altered by the presence of another gas. This effect is seen when oxygen under pressure is passed into a cylinder containing liquid nitrous oxide. Eventually a 50:50 mixture of oxygen and nitrous oxide results; this is Entonox (62.1).

b) F The filling pressure of an Entonox cylinder is 137 atm (62.2).

c) F The mixture is 50:50 oxygen and nitrous oxide (62.3).

d) T Note that the cylinders are French blue and have blue/white shoulders (62.3).

e) F Entonox does not have a boiling point (62.4).

63a) T Atropine is able to cross the blood–brain barrier and thus may be responsible for CNS effects. Atropinic poisoning produces marked delirium and madness (63.1).

b) T Atropine causes relaxation of bronchial smooth muscle with a somewhat greater magnitude in large airways. Anatomical dead space is correspondingly increased (63.1).

c) F As described above (63.1).

d) T Pyrexia may be induced by the inhibition of sweating that atropine causes. This only reaches significance with large doses and paediatric usage of the drug (63.1).

e) T The effects of moderate doses of atropine on heart rate are biphasic, with an initial slowing (thought to be centrally mediated) followed by acceleration (63.1).

64 Hypochromic microcytic anaemia is seen in:
a) folate deficiency
b) pernicious anaemia
c) chronic infection
d) thalassaemia
e) iron deficiency

65 Compared with plasma, CSF has:
a) less protein
b) lower osmolality
c) lower pH
d) lower specific gravity
e) more bicarbonate

66 A patient in respiratory failure secondary to end-stage bronchitis and emphysema may show:
a) elevated CVP
b) papilloedema
c) cyanosis
d) raised Pa_{CO_2}
e) coma

References	
64.1 Souhami	p 1044–1046
65.1 Dunnill	p 85
66.1 Souhami	p 500

64a) F The anaemia of folate deficiency is megaloblastic and macrocytosis the rule. Normocytic hypochromic anaemia may be seen in combined iron and folate deficiency states (64.1).

b) F Pernicious anaemia is a state of vitamin B_{12} deficiency which results in a macrocytic anaemia (64.1).

c) T The anaemia of chronic infection is microcytic and hypochromic (64.1).

d) T Thalassaemia results in a microcytic picture (64.1).

e) T Hypochromia and microcytosis form the classic pattern of iron deficiency anaemia (64.1).

65a) T Total protein in CSF is much lower than plasma (150–400 mg/l) (65.1).

b) F The osmolality of CSF is 306 mosmol/kg which is higher than plasma (65.1).

c) T The pH value for CSF lies between 7.30 and 7.35. Thus CSF is slightly more acidic than plasma (7.32–7.42) (65.1).

d) T The specific gravity of CSF is 1007 as compared with the plasma value of around 1055 (65.1).

e) T The ratio of CSF to plasma bicarbonate is 1.01. This equates to a CSF concentration of 25.1 mmol/l (65.1).

66a) T End-stage pulmonary disease presents a picture of terminal respiratory failure with signs of hypoxia, CO_2 retention and right heart failure. Central venous pressure will generally be elevated (66.1).

b) T Papilloedema and raised intracranial pressure are secondary to CO_2 retention (66.1).

c) T Cyanosis is an obvious corollary of hypoxia (66.1).

d) T As described above (66.1).

e) T In its final stages, respiratory failure leads to confusion and later coma due to the rise in $Pa\text{co}_2$ and fall in $Pa\text{o}_2$ (66.1).

67 Bupivacaine:
a) is an ester
b) is lipid soluble
c) binds to plasma proteins
d) is unaffected by plasma cholinesterase
e) binds to cardiac conducting tissue

68 Complications of supraclavicular brachial plexus block include:
a) pneumothorax
b) Horner's syndrome
c) ptosis
d) convulsions
e) phrenic nerve damage

69 The following factors affect MAC value:
a) premedication
b) age
c) pressure
d) agent
e) sympathetic stimulation

References	
67.1 Dundee	p 283–293
68.1 Synopsis	p 642–648
69.1 Aitkenhead	p 153–155

67a) F Bupivacaine is an amide-linked agent. There are few ester-linked local anaesthetic agents in use today, the majority are amide types (67.1).
   b) T Bupivacaine is relatively highly lipid soluble. Only etidocaine is more so (67.1).
   c) T Bupivacaine is 95% protein bound. This is a higher value than the other commonly used local anaesthetic agents (67.1).
   d) T It is the ester types of local anaesthetic agent which are broken down by cholinesterase, not the amide types (67.1).
   e) T Somewhat debatable. Bupivacaine appears to be more toxic to the heart than other members of the group. Whether this is the consequence of binding to conducting tissue with a high affinity is not clear (67.1).

68a) T Pneumothorax is a constant risk of most approaches to the brachial plexus above the clavicle. It is said that the use of the axillary approach minimises this risk (68.1).
   b) T Horner's syndrome may be seen and is due to blockade of the cervical sympathetic chain (68.1).
   c) T See (b) above. Ptosis is one of the clinical features of Horner's syndrome (68.1).
   d) T As a consequence of the toxicity of the local anaesthetic agent. Intravascular injection will make convulsions more likely (68.1).
   e) T The phrenic nerve is liable to be damaged at the level of the first rib. Accidental blockade of the nerve is more likely than direct damage (68.1).

69a) T MAC value is reduced by the effect of premedication drugs (69.1).
   b) T MAC value is reduced by advancing age. Note that MAC is higher in neonates and infants (69.1).
   c) T MAC values change with ambient pressure. This effect is entirely due to an effect on partial pressure which is related to the potency of anaesthetic agents (69.1).
   d) T MAC is agent specific (69.1).
   e) T Sympathetic stimulation, which may for example be induced by hypercapnia, will cause an increase in MAC value (69.1).

70 Boyle's law relates to:
a) ideal gases
b) pressure and volume
c) change in gas temperature
d) Boyle's bottle
e) volume at constant pressure

71 Static electricity:
a) will be discharged by water on surfaces
b) is decreased by using conductive rubber anaesthetic circuits
c) occurs with non-conducting materials
d) can affect rotameters
e) is reduced by low relative humidity

72 Liver failure may be caused by:
a) paracetamol
b) aspirin
c) death cap fungus
d) paraquat
e) alcohol

References

70.1	Synopsis	p 57–59
70.2	Synopsis	p 18
71.1	Aitkenhead	p 289
71.2	Aitkenhead	p 326
71.3	Aitkenhead	p 296
72.1	Souhami	p 637–644
72.2	Davidson's	p 979

70a) T It may be necessary to return to basic physics for precise definitions. An ideal gas is one which obeys the gas laws under experimental conditions (70.1).

b) T Boyle's law states that at a constant temperature the volume of a given mass of gas varies inversely with the absolute pressure (70.1).

c) F Boyle's law states a constant temperature (70.1).

d) F Robert Boyle was an English chemist (1627–1691) (70.1), who defined the gas law. Henry Edmund Gaskin Boyle was an eminent anaesthetist (1875–1941) who developed the Boyle's machine (70.2). An idea of the order of historical events can be helpful.

e) F Boyle's law is stated in (b) (70.1).

71a) T Moisture allows leakage of static charges along surfaces to earth (71.1).

b) T The rubber used for anaesthetic circuitry is conductive so that static charges can leak to earth (71.2).

c) T Static charges occur on non-conductive material, for example: rubber, plastic, woollen blankets, nylon and terylene (71.1).

d) T Rotameter inaccuracies due to static electricity may be of a magnitude of up to 35%. Static electricity can be reduced by a gold or tin film on the inside of the rotameter tubes (71.3).

e) F Static electricity is reduced by a relative humidity above 50% (71.1).

72a) T Paracetamol is a predictable hepatotoxin causing hepatitis and potential liver failure in overdosage (72.1).

b) T Acute anicteric hepatitis with its attendant sequelae can occur after aspirin treatment especially in children (72.1).

c) T *Amanita phalloides* or death cap fungus, is a poisonous mushroom that can cause fulminant hepatic failure (72.1).

d) T Following ingestion of paraquat multiple organ failure can occur (72.2).

e) T Chronic alcoholic liver disease is the commonest cause of cirrhosis in Europe (72.1).

73 Cooling during surgery can be decreased by:
a) theatre temperature at 20°C
b) space blankets
c) warmed intravenous fluids
d) phenothiazines
e) humidified gases

74 The following drugs are isomeric:
a) halothane
b) enflurane
c) isoflurane
d) methohexitone
e) thiopentone

75 The following drugs are quaternary ammonium compounds:
a) glycopyrronium
b) atropine
c) pancuronium
d) edrophonium
e) nitrous oxide

References

73.1 Aitkenhead	p 325
73.2 Aitkenhead	p 609–610
73.3 BNF	s 4.2.1
73.4 Aitkenhead	p 282
74.1 Dundee	p 112
74.2 Dundee	p 142
75.1 Dundee	p 318
75.2 Dundee	p 305
75.3 Dundee	p 333–337
75.4 Dundee	p 127–131

73a) F An ambient temperature of less than 20°C will allow the development of hypothermia. The recommended temperature in operating theatres is 22–24°C (73.1).
  b) T Loss of heat will be reduced by the use of a space blanket or similar foil cover. The use of metallic covers should be restricted in the presence of diathermy (73.2).
  c) T Intravenous fluids which are warmed prior to their transfusion (peripherally or centrally) will reduce cooling of the patient (73.2).
  d) F Phenothiazines aid cooling due to vasodilatation (via alpha blockade) and CNS depression. The effect is dose related (73.3).
  e) T Humidification of gases conserves heat more effectively than the warming of dry gases (73.4).

74a) F Halothane is not an isomeric structure because it lacks the necessary asymmetrical carbon atom (74.1).
  b) T Enflurane and isoflurane are structural isomers. The atomic composition of both is identical – 3 carbon, 2 hydrogen, 5 fluorine and 1 chlorine – but the chemical formulae differ (74.1).
  c) T See (b) above (74.1).
  d) T Methohexitone has two asymmetrical carbon groups which leads to four potential isomers – alpha and beta, *d* and *l* (74.2).
  e) F Thiopentone is not isomeric (74.2).

75a) T Glycopyrronium is a quaternary ammonium compound. This property is quoted as desirable over atropine because it limits transfer across the blood–brain barrier (75.1).
  b) F Atropine is *d,l* hyoscyamine. There is no quaternary ammonium group in the molecule (75.1).
  c) T Pancuronium is a bisquaternary aminosteroid. It thus has two quaternary nitrogen atoms (75.2).
  d) T Edrophonium is a quaternary ammonium compound, a feature which it shares with other anticholinesterase drugs (excepting physostigmine) (75.3).
  e) F Nitrous oxide is not a quaternary ammonium compound.

76 Aortic incompetence is associated with:
a) ankylosing spondylitis
b) Marfan's syndrome
c) rheumatoid arthritis
d) acromegaly
e) sickle cell disease

77 The following are ethers:
a) halothane
b) methoxyflurane
c) desflurane
d) chloroform
e) sevoflurane

78 Cervical sympathetic trunk sectioning produces:
a) dilated pupils
b) ptosis
c) loss of sweating on the ipsilateral side of the face
d) a dry anterior two thirds of the tongue
e) exopthalmos

References

76.1 Davidson's	p 297
76.2 Davidson's	p 768
76.3 Souhami	p 683
76.4 Davidson's	p 719–721
77.1 Dundee	p 102–113
78.1 Souhami	p 866

76a) T Aortic regurgitation can occur when the first part of the aorta is dilated due to cystic medial necrosis, Marfan's syndrome, ankylosing spondylitis, late syphilis or atheroma (76.1).
   b) T See (a) above (76.1).
   c) T Rare associations that occur with seropositive rheumatoid arthritis are aortic incompetence, coronary artery occlusion, cardiomyopathy and granulomatous lesions that may eventually lead on to heart block (76.2).
   d) F Although associated with hypertension, cardiomyopathy and ischaemic heart disease, acromegaly is not specifically associated with aortic valve disease (76.3).
   e) F Chronic anaemia may result in cardiomegaly but there is no association with aortic valve disease (76.4).

77a) F Ethers are defined by their etheric (C–O–C) bond. Those vapours, such as halothane, which are basically carbon and hydrogen compounds with halogens are classified as hydrocarbons (77.1).
   b) T Methoxyflurane, introduced in 1961 and no longer available, is an halogenated ether (77.1).
   c) T Desflurane is difluromethyl 1-fluro-2,2,2-trifluroethyl ether (77.1).
   d) F Chloroform ($CHCl_3$) is a chlorinated hydrocarbon (77.1).
   e) T Sevoflurane is a recently introduced agent which is a fluorinated ether (77.1).

78a) F Division of the cervical sympathetic trunk produces Horner's syndrome. The effect on the pupil is one of miosis, so the pupil is smaller than the contralateral pupil (78.1).
   b) T Ptosis is a feature of Horner's syndrome (78.1).
   c) T There will be a loss of sweating on the ipsilateral side of the face (78.1).
   d) F The anterior two thirds of the tongue is supplied by the Vth and VIIth cranial nerves (via the chorda tympani).
   e) F Enopthalmos will be seen, not exopthalmos (78.1).

79 Hypokalaemia is associated with:
a) large P waves
b) frusemide
c) steroid therapy
d) paralysis
e) Bartter's syndrome

80 The following drugs demonstrate alpha blockade:
a) prazosin
b) clonidine
c) phenoxybenzamine
d) labetolol
e) phentolamine

81 Insulin:
a) decreases glyconeogenesis
b) increases glycogen production
c) stimulates the conversion of amino acids to protein in the liver
d) raises intracellular potassium concentration
e) is catabolic

References	
79.1 Souhami	p 850–851
80.1 Dundee	p 278–279
80.2 Vickers	p 330–331
80.3 Dundee	p 392–394
81.1 Guyton	p 855–863

79a) F Large T waves are associated with hyperkalaemia. Moderate hyperkalaemia results in peaking of T waves (79.1).
b) T The majority of diuretic drugs cause increased potassium loss in the urine, and frusemide is no exception (79.1).
c) T Hypokalaemia occurs as a result of the mineralocorticoid effect of increased glucocorticoids (79.1).
d) T Generally hypokalaemia results in a level of weakness that falls short of paralysis. The syndrome of familial periodic paralysis <u>does</u> relate hypokalaemia to paralysis, thus the response here should be 'true' (79.1).
e) T Bartter's syndrome is a syndrome of defective reabsorption of chloride in the loop of Henle which leads to general solute loss and secondary hyperaldosteronism (79.1).

80a) T Prazosin is an alpha antagonist at $alpha_1$ post-junctional receptors (80.1).
b) F Clonidine is an alpha <u>agonist</u> with effects at pre- and post-junctional sites (80.2).
c) T Phenoxybenzamine is an alpha blocking agent which acts on $alpha_1$ post-junctional sites (80.1).
d) T Labetalol has both alpha and beta blocking actions. The ratio of alpha to beta effect is 1:10 (80.3).
e) T Phentolamine is an alpha blocking drug acting on $alpha_1$ and $alpha_2$ sites (80.1).

81a) F Insulin causes the formation of glycogen within the liver. It stimulates glyconeogenesis (81.1).
b) T Glycogen production in the liver is increased by a variety of actions. For detail see reference (81.1).
c) T Insulin increases the uptake of amino acids into the liver cells and their subsequent protein synthesis. It is this role of insulin which renders it anabolic (81.1).
d) T Membrane permeability to glucose and potassium is increased by the action of insulin and thus intracellular transfer of potassium from without occurs (81.1).
e) F The reverse is true. See (c) above (81.1).

82 Etomidate:
a) lowers intra-ocular pressure
b) is excreted in the urine
c) causes pituitary suppression
d) causes pain on injection
e) is formulated in propylene glycol

83 One mole of a gas:
a) occupies 22.4 l at room temperature
b) has the same volume for any gas
c) contains Avogadro's number of molecules
d) may be liquefied by compression alone
e) is a gram molecular weight

84 The following are clinical features of rheumatoid arthritis:
a) asymmetrical joint involvement
b) pleural effusion
c) amyloidosis
d) pericarditis
e) coronary arteritis

References		
82.1 Synopsis	p 168–170	
82.2 Aitkenhead	p 185–186	
83.1 Parbrook	p 53–54	
83.2 Parbrook	p 338	
83.3 Parbrook	p 56–59	
84.1 Souhami	p 988–992	

82a) T In premedicated patients intra-ocular pressure is reduced. Cerebral blood flow is also reduced (82.1).

b) F Metabolism occurs in the plasma and the liver, mainly by ester hydrolysis, and the metabolites are excreted in the urine. Around 2% is excreted unchanged (82.2).

c) F Etomidate depresses the synthesis of cortisol at the level of the adrenal gland, so impairing the response to adrenocorticotrophic hormone (ACTH) (82.2).

d) T If a small vein is used injection causes pain in 80% of patients. 10% of patients find injection into a large antecubital fossa vein painful (82.2).

e) T Although soluble in water etomidate is unstable. It is supplied as a clear aqueous solution containing 35% propylene glycol (82.2).

83a) F One mole of gas occupies 22.4 l at standard temperature and pressure (STP) (83.1). Expressed in SI units, STP is 273.15 K (0°C) and 101.325 kPa (83.2).

b) T Avogadro's hypothesis states that equal volumes of gases at the same temperature and pressure contain equal numbers of molecules (83.2).

c) T Avogadro's number is 6.022×10^{23} molecules which are contained in one mole of gas (83.2).

d) F The completion relates to the critical temperature which is defined as the temperature above which a substance cannot be liquefied however much pressure is applied (83.3).

e) T One mole of gas contains the molecular weight of a substance in grams (83.1).

84a) F Characteristically the joint involvement is symmetrical and peripheral. Symmetry of involvement is a distinctive feature of the disease (84.1).

b) T There are several pulmonary features of rheumatoid arthritis. Pleural effusions may be seen (84.1).

c) T Amyloidosis is often seen in accompaniment with chronic disease states. Rheumatoid arthritis is no exception (84.1).

d) T Pericarditis is not common. It is said to be seen in approximately 10% of hospital admissions for the condition and is generally asymptomatic (84.1).

e) T Note that coronary arteritis is rare and usually part of a more generalised arteritis (84.1).

85 Compared with halothane, enflurane has:
a) a higher boiling point
b) a lower SVP
c) a lower MAC
d) a higher molecular weight
e) a lower blood/gas solubility coefficient

86 Alfentanil:
a) is reversed by naloxone
b) has a shorter half-life than fentanyl
c) is excreted by the liver
d) has a large volume of distribution
e) may cause chest wall rigidity

87 Stimulation of the sympathetic system results from:
a) hypoxia
b) hypercapnia
c) hypovolaemia
d) haemorrhage
e) amphetamines

References

85.1 Dunnill   p 7

86.1 Dundee   p 218–227
86.2 Data Sheet   p 659

87.1 Guyton   p 210–202
87.2 Synopsis   p 38–39
87.3 Guyton   p 264–265
87.4 Rang   p 739

85a) T The respective boiling points (atmospheric pressure) are halothane 50°C, enflurane 57°C (85.1).
  b) T At 20°C the respective SVP values are halothane 243 mmHg, enflurane 180 mmHg (85.1).
  c) F The MAC for halothane is 0.8% and that of enflurane 1.7% (85.1).
  d) F The molecular weight of enflurane is 184 Daltons, that of halothane 197 Daltons (85.1).
  e) T The blood gas solubility coefficient of enflurane is 1.9 while the corresponding value for halothane is 2.5 (85.1).

86a) T Naloxone will reverse the effect of any opioid agonist agent (86.1).
  b) T The terminal half-life of alfentanil is 1.5 h. The terminal half life for fentanyl is 3–4 h (86.1).
  c) T Hepatic clearance is the major route of excretion of the drug (86.1).
  d) F The volume of distribution of alfentanil is low, of the order of 1 l/kg. Most of the other commonly used opioid drugs have a volume of distribution around a value of 6 l/kg (86.1).
  e) T The so called 'wooden chest' rigidity is less common than with fentanyl but may occur after the use of alfentanil also (86.2).

87a) T When hypoxia develops in the brain stem the vasomotor centre responds in such a way as to become excited and increase its discharge. The result is a strong increase in general sympathetic tone (87.1).
  b) T Hypercapnia is a potent stimulator of sympatho-adrenal activity (87.2).
  c) T For practical purposes here hypovolaemia and haemorrhage may be considered together. In both situations a fall in circulating volume stimulates a response from the baroreceptors and low pressure receptors which results in widespread sympatho-adrenal stimulation (87.3).
  d) T See (c) above (87.3).
  e) T Amphetamines have peripheral alpha and beta actions which are analogous to indirectly acting sympathomimetic agents. The net result is an increase in sympathetic tone (87.4).

88 Oxygen:
a) is stored in cylinders at 137 kPa when full
b) is stored in black cylinders
c) has a critical temperature of 118°C
d) is liquid in the cylinder
e) supports combustion

89 Carbon dioxide:
a) is stored in gaseous form
b) is stored in green cylinders
c) is stored at a pressure of 200 atm
d) supports combustion
e) has a critical temperature of 31°C

90 With respect to the scavenging of gases and vapours:
a) a large pressure gradient is used
b) scavenging is always passive
c) sub-atmospheric pressures are used
d) a pressure relief valve is required
e) passive systems are affected by wind

References	
88.1 Ward	p 32–35
89.1 Ward	p 32–35
90.1 Ward	p 280–285

88a) F Oxygen is stored in cylinders at a pressure of 137×10^3 kPa. Be scrupulously careful over the units in this type of question (88.1).
  b) T To be strictly accurate, the cylinders are black but the shoulders are coloured white (88.1).
  c) F The critical temperature of oxygen is <u>minus</u> 118°C (88.1).
  d) F Within the cylinder oxygen is in gaseous form (88.1).
  e) T This is very obvious (88.1).

89a) F Carbon dioxide is in liquid physical state within the cylinder (89.1).
  b) F The true colour of carbon dioxide cylinders is grey (89.1).
  c) F Carbon dioxide is stored at a pressure of 50 atmospheres or 5×10^3 kPa when full (89.1).
  d) F Combustion is not supported (89.1). Carbon dioxide gas is used as a fire extinguisher (89.1).
  e) T The critical temperature of carbon dioxide is 31°C (89.1).

90a) F In the design of scavenging systems it is important that a small pressure gradient exists between patient circuit and scavenging pipe work (90.1).
  b) F Scavenging systems may be passive (where the patient's work of exhalation drives gas) or active (where a sub-atmospheric pressure is used to remove gas from the patient valve) (90.1).
  c) T As described above (90.1).
  d) T In scavenging systems two safeguards are used. Within the reservoir of the scavenging system a valve is installed to allow escape of gas if a pressure build-up occurs. The second safety device is a valve which will open at a sub-atmospheric pressure of 0.5 cmH_2O to admit air if the demand of the extraction system becomes excessive (90.1).
  e) T Passive systems are usually simply vented to the exterior and are therefore affected by wind speed and direction (90.1).

91 Propranolol:
   a) is a membrane stabiliser
   b) can be given orally or intravenously
   c) should be avoided in asthmatic patients
   d) should be avoided in patients on disopyramide
   e) should be avoided in hypokalaemic states

92 Convulsions can be caused by:
   a) hypoxia
   b) enflurane
   c) bupivacaine
   d) halothane
   e) methohexitone

93 The jugular venous pulse:
   a) has a height which reflects central venous pressure
   b) should be measured with a patient at 30°
   c) has an accentuated 'a' wave in atrial fibrillation
   d) shows giant 'v' waves in tricuspid regurgitation
   e) is normally less than 3 cm above the sternal angle

References

91.1 Dundee		p 403–408
91.2 Dundee		p 362
92.1 Synopsis		p 276–277
93.1 Souhami		p 337–338

91a) T Propranolol has membrane stabilising properties, is a potent local anaesthetic and is a class II anti-arrhythmic agent by the Vaughan-Williams classification (91.1).

b) T Propranolol is rapidly and fully absorbed by mouth but there is then a marked first pass effect due to liver metabolism. Bioavailability is about 10–30%. Hence the difference between oral and intravenous doses (91.1).

c) T Beta blocking drugs, particularly non-selective ones, produce a rise in airways resistance (91.1).

d) F Caution should be exercised when propranolol is given in combination with class I anti-arrythmics such as disopyramide or verapamil and when changing treatment from clonidine (91.1).

e) F Do not confuse precautions of propranolol treatment with precautions of digoxin therapy (91.2).

92a) T Hypoxia can cause convulsions (92.1).

b) T Enflurane and methohexitone cause increased activity on EEG, and epileptiform convulsions have been reported (92.1).

c) T Convulsions occur secondary to local anaesthetic drug toxicity (92.1).

d) F Severe myoclonus may be confused with convulsions (92.1).

e) T Convulsions have been reported due to methohexitone (92.1).

93a) T The height of the jugular venous pressure (JVP) is dependent on central venous pressure (93.1).

b) F The patient should be reclining at 45° on a bed with head supported (93.1).

c) F The 'a' wave is generated by atrial systole, it is therefore absent in atrial fibrillation (93.1).

d) T Regurgitation through the tricuspid valve results in a giant 'v' wave (otherwise termed 's' wave) with a rapid descent (93.1).

e) T Anaesthetists usually work with central venous pressure rather than the less precise jugular venous pressure. A normal JVP is less than 3 cm vertically above the sternal angle (93.1).

---

94 Bowel activity is increased by:
a) atropine
b) neostigmine
c) mechanical distension
d) vagal stimulation
e) epidural anaesthesia

---

95 Acute intestinal obstruction:
a) carries an increased risk of aspiration on induction
b) will be accompanied by hypovolaemia
c) is accompanied by decreased serum chloride
d) is accompanied by decreased serum potassium
e) requires a nasogastric tube in place during induction of anaesthesia

---

96 Acute intermittent porphyria is a contraindication to the use of:
a) methohexitone
b) morphine
c) pentazocine
d) ketamine
e) etomidate

References	
94.1 Dundee	p 320
94.2 Dundee	p 335
94.3 Guyton	p 703
94.4 Guyton	p 672–673
94.5 Synopsis	p 702
95.1 Aitkenhead	p 659
95.2 Synopsis	p 444–446
96.1 Synopsis	p 393–394

94a) F Atropine reduces the frequency and amplitude of contractions in all parts of the gastro-intestinal tract (94.1).
b) T The motility of both large and small bowel is increased by neostigmine (94.2).
c) T Mechanical distension of any part of the bowel excites increased peristalsis (94.3).
d) T The action of the vagus is to increase peristalsis in the gastrointestinal tract (94.3).
e) F The action of both epidural and subarachnoid anaesthesia is to provide sympathetic ablation to the affected segments. As the sympathetic supply to the bowel is inhibitory, the small bowel will become contracted. Sphincters are relaxed and peristalsis, although active, is no more than normal (94.5).

95a) T In acute intestinal obstruction there is an increased risk of aspiration of gastric contents (95.1).
b) T Fluid and electrolyte depletion lead to hypovolaemia (95.1).
c) T Serum chloride is usually low. This occurs in part from direct loss due to vomiting, and secondarily from alkalosis which exacerbates the situation (95.2).
d) T Serum potassium will usually be low. This situation pertains even when considering the artificial elevation of serum biochemical values which is seen in dehydration (95.2).
e) F It is recommended by most sources that a nasogastric tube should be aspirated and then withdrawn. Hopefully this will remove the risk of aspiration around the tube itself (95.2).

96a) T All barbiturates are contraindicated in porphyric states, as the enzyme delta-ALA-synthetase is stimulated thus increasing the rate of formation of porphobilinogens (96.1).
b) F Morphine has been recommended for use in porphyrias (96.1).
c) T Pentazocine should be avoided (96.1).
d) F Ketamine appears to be safe to use as an intravenous induction agent (96.1).
e) F Etomidate has been recommended for use in porphyrias when an intravenous induction is necessary (96.1). There remains residual uncertainty over the desirability of etomidate for patients with porphyria, due to conflicting animal studies.

97 Sulphonylureas:
a) are antagonised by thiazide diuretics
b) promote pancreatic beta cells to release insulin
c) are protein bound
d) include metoclopramide
e) have no extrapancreatic action

98 Tolbutamide:
a) can be used in renal impairment
b) is short acting
c) can be used in porphyria
d) can cause thrombocytopenia
e) has a half-life of 10 h

99 In the Valsalva manoeuvre:
a) there is an increase in intrathoracic pressure
b) there is a decrease in heart rate
c) there is an increase in cardiac output
d) peripheral resistance falls
e) pulse pressure increases

References

97.1	BNF	Appendix 1
97.2	BNF	s 6.1.2.1
97.3	Dundee	p 500
97.4	BNF	s 4.6
98.1	BNF	s 6.1.2.1
98.2	Dundee	p 500
99.1	Ganong	p 558

97a) T The hypoglycaemic effect of sulphonylureas is antagonised by loop and thiazide diuretics (97.1).
   b) T The main action of sulphonylurea drugs is to augment insulin secretion, via residual pancreatic beta cell activity (97.2).
   c) T Sulphonylureas are carried bound to protein and their action may be potentiated by other protein-bound drugs (97.3).
   d) F Metoclopramide is an antiemetic unrelated to sulphonylureas (97.4).
   e) T Extrapancreatic actions are seen during long-term administration of sulphonylureas (97.2).

98a) T Tolbutamide may be used in renal impairment (98.1) as the metabolism is hepatic (98.2).
   b) T The duration of action is short with a half-life of 5 h (98.2).
   c) F Sulphonylureas should be avoided in porphyrias (98.1).
   d) T Blood disorders occur infrequently. These may include thrombocytopaenia, agranulocytosis and aplastic anaemia (98.1).
   e) F The half-life is 5 h (98.2). Do not guess.

99a) T Intrathoracic pressure increases with the onset of straining (99.1).
   b) F There is a rise in heart rate to compensate for the fall in blood pressure (99.1).
   c) F The increase in intrathoracic pressure causes venous compression and a reduction in venous return, resulting in a fall in cardiac output (99.1).
   d) F There is a rise in peripheral resistance which is a compensation for the falling blood pressure (99.1).
   e) F Pulse pressure and blood pressure fall as venous return is lost (99.1).

100 With respect to ketamine:
  a) dreams are worse in children
  b) morphine premedication will reduce the incidence of dreams
  c) diazepam will reduce the incidence of dreams
  d) a quiet recovery will reduce the incidence of dreams
  e) incidence of dreams diminishes with daily ketamine treatment

101 In the first 24 hours after surgery:
  a) urine output is high
  b) sodium loss is increased
  c) potassium loss is increased
  d) ADH secretion falls
  e) plasma osmolality is unchanged

102 Chlorpromazine:
  a) is an alpha blocker
  b) is a beta blocker
  c) may induce hypothermia
  d) is a butyrophenone
  e) may cause sedation

References	
100.1 Dundee	p 167–168
101.1 Synopsis 10e	p 39–40
101.2 Aitkenhead	p 393–403
102.1 Synopsis 10e	p 246–247

100a) F Although there is uncertainty over the issue, it is generally held that neither emergence delirium nor excessively vivid dreams occur in young children (100.1).

  b) T The incidence of unpleasant dreams is markedly reduced by opioid premedication (100.1).

  c) T Diazepam is thought to reduce the incidence of dreams after ketamine due to its combined sedative and amnesic properties (100.1).

  d) T The less stimulation a patient receives during the recovery period, the less dreams will occur (100.1).

  e) T Experience with burned patients suggests that the incidence of dreams diminishes with repeat exposure (100.1).

101a) F The response to surgery and trauma is a classic stress response. Part of this picture is an increase in circulating ADH, which leads to a fall in urine output and decreased serum osmolality (101.1, 101.2).

  b) F In the first 24 hours sodium loss is reduced due to an increase in aldosterone (101.1).

  c) T Tissue damage and catabolism lead to an increased loss of potassium (101.2).

  d) F ADH secretion is increased. See (a) above (101.1).

  e) F Usually osmolality will fall due to the action of ADH. Aldosterone secretion which causes retention of sodium will mitigate against this (101.2).

102a) T Chlorpromazine has alpha blocking activity but this is not of great magnitude (102.1).

  b) T Chlorpromazine is a weak beta blocker (102.1).

  c) T The suppression of shivering combined with vasodilation may lead to hypothermia (102.1).

  d) F Chlorpromazine is not a butyrophenone. It is a member of the phenothiazine family (102.1).

  e) T The drug is extremely sedative. This is its major use in psychiatric patients (102.1).

103 With regard to cardiopulmonary resuscitation (CPR):
a) survival is more likely if the rhythm is ventricular fibrillation
b) chest compressions should be 100/min
c) for two resuscitators the ventilation/compression ratio should be 10:1
d) for a single resuscitator the ventilation/compression ratio should be 15:2
e) resuscitation bags usually deliver high concentrations of oxygen

104 In the burned patient:
a) suxamethonium should not be used
b) cyanide poisoning may be seen
c) colloid only should be transfused
d) respiratory distress syndrome may develop
e) laryngeal oedema is seen

105 Methohexitone:
a) causes seizures
b) has a pKa of 8.9
c) is alkaline in solution
d) causes pain on injection in 50% of patients
e) is used as a 10% solution

References	
103.1 BMJ (1989) 299	p 442–444
104.1 Mason	p 38–41
105.1 Synopsis	p 276
105.2 Dundee	p 137–154
105.3 Synopsis	p 167–168

103a) T In guidelines issued by the Resuscitation Council (UK) it is stated that survival from cardiac arrest is optimal when the rhythm preceding collapse is ventricular fibrillation (103.1).

b) F To provide adequate output while avoiding fatigue a rate of 60–80/min is recommended (103.1).

c) F The correct ratio is 5:1 (103.1).

d) T 15:2 is recommended for single person techniques (103.1).

e) F Resuscitation bags <u>can</u> deliver high concentrations of oxygen but <u>only</u> if an entrainment reservoir is used (103.1).

104a) F Suxamethonium is only contraindicated between the 20th and 60th day after injury due to the excessive release of potassium which may occur (104.1).

b) T Cyanide poisoning may accompany burns (as may carbon monoxide poisoning) (104.1). This is often due to the combustion of furnishing foam cushions which may yield cyanide gas.

c) F The ideal situation is a mix of colloid and crystalloid solutions (104.1).

d) T Respiratory distress syndrome may occur as late as the fourth day after injury (104.1).

e) T Laryngeal oedema is usually secondary to direct heat or smoke injury (104.1).

105a) T Epileptiform seizures have been reported after methohexitone (105.1). Focal EEG discharge is increased.

b) F The pKa of methohexitone is 8.1 (105.2).

c) T The pH of a prepared methohexitone solution suitable for clinical use is 11.1 (105.3).

d) F The incidence of pain on injection is 25–30% (105.1).

e) F Methohexitone is used as a 1% solution (105.3).

106 With respect to total intravenous anaesthesia:
   a) ketamine is suitable
   b) it is suitable for anaesthesia involving paralysis and IPPV
   c) MIR is equivalent to MAC
   d) it is contraindicated in surgery of long duration
   e) a bolus dose is used to start anaesthesia

107 Reduction of dislocated shoulder can be carried out under:
   a) Bier's block
   b) axillary block
   c) interscalene block
   d) suprascapular nerve block
   e) general anaesthesia

108 End tidal CO$_2$:
   a) shows a 0.7 kPa gradient against arterial
   b) is measured by ultraviolet absorption spectrophotometry
   c) will fall in malignant hyperpyrexia
   d) rises during hypoventilation
   e) rises during pulmonary embolism

References	
106.1 Aitkenhead	p 188–189
107.1 Synopsis	p 642–650
107.2 Aitkenhead	p 494
108.1 Aitkenhead	p 379-380

106a) F Drugs for total intravenous anaesthesia (TIVA) should be metabolised and eliminated rapidly to avoid accumulation. At present propofol is the only realistic contender (106.1).

b) T Although the technique is used in paralysed patients there is a risk of awareness if inadequate doses are used (106.1).

c) T Minimal infusion rate (MIR) is defined as the rate of infusion which produces loss of motor response to surgical stimulation in 50% of patients. It is equivalent to the effective dose in 50% of the population (ED_{50}) or the minimum alveolar concentration for volatile agents (MAC) (106.1).

d) F The use of TIVA in operations longer than 8 h avoids depression of bone marrow function by prolonged use of nitrous oxide (106.1). Note that TIVA has been advocated when accompanied by an air-oxygen mixture rather than nitrous oxide.

e) T A bolus dose or high infusion rate is used initially to achieve an adequate blood concentration (106.1).

107a) F Bier's block or intravenous regional anaesthesia (IVRA) produces analgesia below the cuff on the upper arm. There is no analgesia of the shoulder joint (107.1).

b) F The axillary approach to the brachial plexus is not satisfactory for reduction of dislocated shoulder (107.1).

c) T The interscalene approach to the brachial plexus is satisfactory for reduction of a dislocated shoulder (107.1).

d) F Suprascapular nerve block provides analgesia of the shoulder joint (including rotator cuff) but not for the overlying skin. It is a satisfactory technique for chronic pain relief but not for surgery. The retention of muscle tone in the surrounding muscles (supraspinatus excluded) makes reduction impossible (107.1).

e) T As reduction of dislocated shoulder is often performed in accident and emergency departments care should be taken concerning starvation and preparation of the patient (107.2).

108a) T In patients with no significant pulmonary disease the normal Pa_{CO_2}–Pe_{CO_2} gradient is approximately 0.7 kPa (108.1).

b) F Carbon dioxide concentration is measured by infrared absorption spectrophotometry (108.1).

c) F The increase in muscle metabolism produces a rise in carbon dioxide with a rise in end tidal carbon dioxide (108.1).

d) T End tidal carbon dioxide can be used as a method of monitoring adequate ventilation (108.1).

e) F A sudden decrease in end tidal carbon dioxide will occur with air, fat or thrombotic pulmonary embolism (108.1).

109 A rise in temperature:
  a) increases liquid vaporisation
  b) can be measured by a Bourdon gauge
  c) increases the amount of gas dissolved in a liquid
  d) moves the oxyhaemoglobin saturation curve to the left
  e) is related to saturated vapour pressure

110 The rate of gas diffusion through a membrane is proportional to:
  a) pressure
  b) membrane surface area
  c) membrane thickness
  d) gas molecular weight
  e) gas solubility

111 Enflurane:
  a) depresses respiratory rate
  b) has a higher oil/gas coefficient than halothane
  c) depresses the myocardium
  d) the MAC is lower than halothane
  e) has a lower boiling point than halothane

References
109.1 Aitkenhead   p 282
109.2 Parbrook   p 115
109.3 Parbrook   p 78
109.4 Aitkenhead   p 39
109.5 Parbrook   p 137–140

110.1 West   p 21–22

111.1 Aitkenhead   p 163–164
111.2 Aitkenhead   p 723

109a) T Increasing the temperature of a liquid results in an increase in the kinetic energy of molecules and a greater number of molecules escape to become vapour (109.1).

b) T The Bourdon gauge measures pressure but with a suitable sensor or transducer, temperature may be converted to a pressure change (109.2).

c) F As temperature rises less gas dissolves in a liquid (109.3).

d) F A rise in temperature will move the oxyhaemoglobin saturation curve to the right (109.4).

e) T There is an increase in vapour pressure with an increase in temperature in a non-linear fashion (109.5).

110a) T Fick's law states that the rate of diffusion of a substance across unit area is proportional to the concentration gradient. In the gas phase tension or partial pressure can replace the term concentration gradient (110.1).

b) T Rate of gas diffusion is proportional to the membrane surface area (110.1).

c) F Rate of gas diffusion is <u>inversely</u> proportional to the membrane thickness (110.1).

d) F Rate of diffusion is inversely proportional to the square root of the molecular weight of the gas (110.1).

e) T Rate of diffusion is proportional to gas solubility (110.1).

111a) F There is an increase in respiratory rate with a reduction in tidal volume resulting in depression of alveolar ventilation (111.1).

b) F The oil/gas solubility coefficient for enflurane is 98 and that for halothane is 220 (111.2).

c) T The myocardial depression is dose dependent and depression of cardiac output results (111.1).

d) F The MAC of enflurane is 1.68 and that of halothane is 0.8 (111.2).

e) F The boiling point of enflurane is 56°C and that of halothane is 50°C (111.2).

112 The following drugs relax skeletal muscle:
a) baclofen
b) diazepam
c) gallamine
d) chlorpromazine
e) ketamine

113 In disseminated intravascular coagulation (DIC):
a) Gram-negative septicaemia is a predisposing factor
b) fibrinolysis is reduced
c) heparin is contraindicated
d) thrombocytopenia occurs
e) treatment with fresh frozen plasma is appropriate

114 Dobutamine:
a) is a strong chronotropic agent
b) is isomeric
c) does not exhibit tolerance
d) increases systemic vascular resistance
e) is harmless if peripheral extravasation occurs

References	
112.1 BNF	s 10.2.2
112.2 BNF	s 15.1.5
112.3 Dundee	p 196
112.4 Dundee	p 166
113.1 Mason	p 462–463
114.1 Dundee	p 352–354

112a) T Baclofen, a derivative of GABA, is used in the treatment of spasticity. A generalised reduction in muscle tone is seen (112.1).
  b) T Diazepam causes relaxation of skeletal muscle. It is particularly useful in the relief of acute muscle spasm (112.1).
  c) T Gallamine is a little used agent which belongs to the non-depolarising muscle relaxants. Excretion of the drug is almost exclusively renal (112.2).
  d) T Chlorpromazine has a variety of clinical effects. It is said to relax skeletal muscle in some spasticity states. Convulsions may also occur. The response is the authors' choice (112.3).
  e) F The effect of ketamine on skeletal muscle is to increase tone rather than to reduce it. Tonic-clonic movements are frequent during anaesthesia with ketamine as sole agent (112.4).

113a) T Gram-negative septicaemia predisposes to DIC (113.1).
  b) F Fibrinolysis is increased. There is evidence of generalised consumption of clotting factors (113.1).
  c) F Note that although heparin is not contraindicated there is considerable controversy over the precise role of heparin in DIC. At present heparin is not recommended (113.1).
  d) T Thrombocytopenia is part of the generalised consumptive process that is seen (113.1).
  e) T Fresh frozen plasma will be useful in treatment due to its high content of clotting factors (113.1).

114a) F Dobutamine is a selective beta$_1$ receptor agonist (although there may be other receptor effects); it produces a strong positive inotropic effect with little chronotropy (114.1).
  b) T The commercial preparation of dobutamine is racemic and the difference in action of the isomers is small (114.1).
  c) F When infusion is continued for more than 48-72 h tolerance may be seen. This can be overcome by an increase in infusion rate (114.1).
  d) F Systemic vascular resistance may not change or may be moderately decreased (114.1).
  e) F Skin necrosis and sloughing due to extravasation have been reported. Administration is possible via a peripheral vein although the central route is preferred (114.1).

---

115 The following features are seen in Parkinson's disease:
a) intention tremor
b) hyperkinesia
c) rigidity
d) greasy skin
e) macrographia

---

116 Features of IIIrd cranial nerve palsy include:
a) upward and outward deviation of the ipsilateral eye
b) pupillary constriction
c) ptosis
d) paralysis of the lateral rectus muscle
e) inability to abduct the ipsilateral eye

---

117 In ulnar nerve injury at the elbow:
a) wrist drop will result
b) ring and little fingers are clawed
c) simian deformity occurs
d) there is sensory loss over the dorsum of the hand
e) there is thenar eminence wasting

References

115.1 Davidson's   p 868–869

116.1 Souhami   p 867

117.1 Macleod   p 266–267

115a) F The tremor of Parkinson's disease is classically seen at rest, in contrast to the intention tremor of cerebellar disease (115.1).
  b) F Hypokinesia is the rule. The classic triad of symptoms in Parkinson's disease is tremor, rigidity and hypokinesia (115.1).
  c) T See (b) above (115.1).
  d) T One of the general physical abnormalities which are seen in Parkinsonism is greasy skin, the exact cause of which is poorly understood (115.1).
  e) F Macrographia (large writing) is not seen. It is micrographia which is a feature of Parkinsonism (115.1).

116a) F IIIrd cranial nerve palsy leads to outward and downward deviation of the eye on the affected side (116.1).
  b) F Provided the pupillary constrictor fibres are affected by the lesion there will be pupillary dilatation (116.1).
  c) T Ptosis is normally seen (116.1).
  d) F Paralysis of the lateral rectus muscle is the result of a lesion of the VIth (abducent) cranial nerve (116.1).
  e) F Failure of abduction of the ipsilateral eye is the result of denervation of the lateral rectus muscle which is supplied by the VIth cranial nerve (116.1).

117a) F Wrist drop results from damage to the radial nerve which supplies the wrist and finger extensors (117.1).
  b) T The ulnar nerve supplies all the small muscles of the hand except the short flexor, abductor and opponents of the thumb, and lumbricals to the index and sometimes middle finger. Clawing is the result of unopposed action of the long flexors and extensors (117.1).
  c) F Simian deformity is the flat ape-like position of the thumb resulting from thenar eminence wasting which occurs after median nerve lesions (117.1).
  d) F An ulnar nerve injury results in loss of sensation on the ulnar border of the hand (117.1).
  e) F Thenar eminence wasting results from median nerve injuries (117.1).

118 Concerning anaesthetic gas cylinders:
a) they are manufactured from carbon steel
b) oxygen is stored as a liquid in cylinders
c) filling ratio is higher in tropical climates
d) carbon dioxide cylinders should be mounted vertically
e) the tare weight is the weight of a full cylinder

119 The following are used in Rapid Sequence Induction:
a) non-depolarising relaxants
b) cricoid pressure
c) nasogastric tube
d) pre-oxygenation
e) suxamethonium

120 Drugs which trigger malignant hyperpyrexia include:
a) suxamethonium
b) pancuronium
c) lignocaine
d) thiopentone
e) halothane

References	
118.1 Ward	p 32–33
119.1 Miller	p 1310–1311
120.1 Synopsis	p 284–286

118a) F Modern gas cylinders are constructed from molybdenum steel which allows thinner walls because of its great strength (118.1).

   b) F Oxygen is stored in cylinders as compressed gas (118.1).

   c) F Filling ratio (weight of substance in the cylinder compared to the weight of water the cylinder could hold) is less in tropical climates, 0.67 compared to 0.75 in temperate climates (118.1).

   d) T Any cylinder which contains liquid should be kept vertical. This applies to nitrous oxide and cylcopropane in addition to carbon dioxide (118.1).

   e) F Tare weight is the weight of an empty cylinder (118.1).

119a) F Rapid sequence induction requires the use of fast-acting, effective muscle relaxants. These are by definition depolarising drugs and to all intents and purposes this means suxamethonium. Note that some parties advocate the use of vecuronium after priming (119.1).

   b) T Cricoid pressure is an essential part of rapid sequence induction (119.1).

   c) F Although the use of a nasogastric tube is advocated in cases of intestinal obstruction its presence makes cricoid pressure ineffective (119.1).

   d) T Pre-oxygenation for 2 min is recommended (119.1).

   e) T See (a) above (119.1).

120a) T Suxamethonium and halothane are the two most commonly implicated anaesthetic agents in malignant hyperpyrexia (MH) (120.1).

   b) F Pancuronium is recommended as a relaxant in suspected cases of MH (120.1).

   c) T Lignocaine is implicated as a trigger agent along with all amide local anaesthetic agents (120.1).

   d) F The anaesthetic drugs which are considered safe are thiopentone, opioids, diazepam, pancuronium and possibly nitrous oxide (120.1).

   e) T Halothane has frequently been cited as a trigger agent in malignant hyperpyrexia (120.1).

121 When a patient given thiopentone and suxamethonium develops muscle rigidity, this may be due to:
a) low plasma cholinesterase
b) malignant hyperpyrexia
c) myotonica congenita
d) dystrophia myotonia
e) familial periodic paralysis

122 A patient who cannot breathe one hour after 50 mg of suxamethonium may:
a) have homozygous atypical gene for plasma cholinesterase
b) have malignant hyperpyrexia
c) have liver disease
d) require stored blood to raise plasma cholinesterase
e) require intravenous cholinesterase

123 Methaemoglobinaemia can be:
a) caused by prilocaine
b) caused by carbon monoxide poisoning
c) caused by trichloroethylene
d) treated with methylene blue
e) treated with ascorbic acid

References	
121.1 Mason	p 225–228
121.2 Mason	p 169–173
121.3 Mason	p 81–83
121.4 Mason	p 103–105
122.1 Mason	p 225–228
122.2 Mason	p 169–173
123.1 Synopsis	p 389
123.2 Souhami	p 59–60
123.3 Synopsis 10e	p 182–185

121a) F The combination of suxamethonium and a low plasma cholinesterase results in prolongation of muscle paralysis without rigidity (121.1).
  b) T Failure of muscle to relax after suxamethonium may be the first indication of malignant hyperpyrexia in an unknown case. Thiopentone is considered to be safe to use (121.2).
  c) T Myotonia is a persistence of muscle contraction beyond the duration of the voluntary effort or duration. In myotonia congenita, suxamethonium can produce a prolonged contraction which outlasts the duration of effect of the drug (121.3).
  d) T Suxamethonium has similar effects in dystrophia myotonica to those described above in myotonia congenita (121.3).
  e) F General anaesthesia may precipitate paralysis in this condition (121.4).

122a) T The homozygous atypical gene group constitutes the majority of suxamethonium-sensitive patients (122.1).
  b) F In malignant hyperpyrexia tachypnoea occurs and in paralysed patients there is an increased requirement for relaxant drugs (122.2).
  c) T Low levels of plasma cholinesterase have been reported in: severe liver disease, malnutrition, renal failure, malignant disease, tetanus, Huntingdon's chorea and collagen disorders (122.1).
  d) F Treatment consists of ventilation and sedation until muscle power returns. Stored blood contains very little plasma cholinesterase (122.1).
  e) F Fresh frozen plasma has been advocated but the risks of HIV (human immunodeficiency virus) may now outweigh the benefits (122.1).

123a) T Methaemoglobinaemia can be idiopathic or secondary to agents such as nitrites, sulphonamides, phenacetin and prilocaine (123.1).
  b) F Carbon monoxide poisoning results in the formation of carboxyhaemoglobin which has a characteristic cherry red colour (123.2).
  c) F Trichloroethylene is not responsible for methaemoglobinaemia formation (123.3).
  d) T Intravenous injection of 1% methylene blue (1–2 mg/kg given over 5 min) converts methaemoglobin to normal haemoglobin (123.1).
  e) T Methaemoglobin can be reconverted to haemoglobin by reducing agents such as ascorbic acid, glutathione and methylene blue (123.1).

124 The following may be seen after supraclavicular brachial plexus block:
a) enopthalmos
b) intravascular injection
c) spread of local anaesthetic to the subarachnoid space
d) elevated hemi-diaphragm
e) pleural puncture

125 Horner's Syndrome:
a) is a lesion of the cervical parasympathetic system
b) results in miosis
c) results in ptosis
d) causes enopthalmos
e) causes increased sweating

126 The femoral nerve:
a) lies medial to the femoral artery
b) may supply part of the foot
c) block requires less than 5 ml of local anaesthetic
d) block is suitable for malleolar surgery
e) block is suitable for knee surgery

References	
124.1 Synopsis	p 642–648
125.1 Souhami	p 866
126.1 Aitkenhead	p 481–482

124a) T A sympathetic block leading to Horner's syndrome is relatively common; a description of Horner's syndrome can be found below. Enopthalmos is one of the features (124.1).

b) T A perivascular approach occasionally results in vascular puncture although this should not be allowed to lead to injection (124.1).

c) T Subarachnoid or extradural spread of local anaesthetic is possible (124.1).

d) T Often asymptomatic, phrenic nerve paralysis is nonetheless common and this leads to elevation of the corresponding hemi-diaphragm (124.1).

e) T Although always present, the risk of pneumothorax decreases with experience of the anaesthetist (124.1). The apical dome of the pleura is vulnerable from this approach to the brachial plexus.

125a) F Horner's syndrome is the result of a lesion in sympathetic fibres (125.1).

b) T Miosis is constriction of the pupil (125.1).

c) T Ptosis is a feature of Horner's syndrome (125.1).

d) T Enopthalmos, the abnormal retraction of the eye into its socket, is due to the sympathetic nerve lesion (125.1).

e) F There is loss of sweating on the ipsilateral side of the face (125.1).

126a) F The femoral nerve lies 2–3 cm lateral to and slightly deeper than the femoral artery (126.1).

b) T The femoral nerve terminates as the saphenous nerve, which supplies the medial side of the calf as far as the medial malleolus and sometimes the medial side of the dorsum of the foot (126.1).

c) F 10–15 ml of solution is the recommended volume (126.1).

d) F Femoral nerve block is inadequate for surgery to the foot or ankle as its supply to this area is variable (126.1).

e) T Femoral nerve block alone may be adequate for knee surgery (126.1).

127 Thiazide diuretics may cause:
a) hyponatraemia
b) hypokalaemic alkalosis
c) hyperuricaemia
d) hyperchloraemia
e) hyperglycaemia

128 Deep vein thrombosis is associated with:
a) anaemia
b) bed rest
c) treatment with ancrod
d) malignancy
e) increased age

129 The following may result in barotrauma:
a) PEEP
b) nitrous oxide
c) poor lung compliance
d) IPPV
e) high airway pressures

References		
127.1 BNF		s 2.2.1
128.1 Davidson's		p 338–339
128.2 BNF		s 2.8.1
129.1 Aitkenhead		p 686
129.2 Aitkenhead		p 500

127a) T Bendrofluazide is an example of a thiazide diuretic. Hyponatraemia, hypokalaemia, hypomagnesaemia and hypochloraemia may occur during treatment (127.1).
  b) F The alkalosis is due to hypochloraemia (127.1).
  c) T Hyperuricaemia, hypercalcaemia and hyperglycaemia are all side effects. Hyperuricaemia may lead to gout (127.1).
  d) F Hypochloraemia is seen during thiazide therapy (127.1).
  e) T Hyperglycaemia can occur (127.1).

128a) F Polycythaemia is a predisposing factor to the development of deep vein thrombosis (DVT) (128.1).
  b) T Immobility due to bed rest, surgery or limb paralysis can result in DVT (128.1).
  c) T Ancrod is an anticoagulant occasionally used for the treatment of DVT and in the prevention of post-operative thrombosis. The drug is obtained from an extract of Malaysian pit viper venom. It reduces plasma fibrinogen by cleavage of fibrin (128.2).
  d) T Malignancy, particularly pelvic, increases the incidence of DVT (128.1).
  e) T Increasing age increases the risk of DVT (128.1).

129a) T The application of positive end expiratory pressure (PEEP) can cause or exaggerate barotrauma (129.1).
  b) F Nitrous oxide per se will not cause barotrauma but if used in patients with closed air spaces, such as a pneumothorax, there will be an increase in pressure within the space (129.2).
  c) T Poor lung compliance will result in high airway pressures during artificial ventilation of the lungs (129.1).
  d) T Intermittent positive pressure ventilation (IPPV) can cause barotrauma even without PEEP or high airway pressures (129.1).
  c) T High airway pressures result in barotrauma (129.1).

130 Gastric motility may be decreased by:
a) atropine
b) morphine
c) neostigmine
d) halothane
e) metoclopramide

131 Lignocaine:
a) does not cross the placenta
b) is lipid soluble
c) can be used to treat convulsions
d) demonstrates tachyphylaxis during continuous epidural infusion
e) is an amide

132 In Chronic Obstructive Pulmonary Disease (COPD):
a) there must be a life-long history of acute attacks of bronchitis
b) FEV_1/FVC is normal
c) residual volume increases
d) peak expiratory flow increases
e) airway resistance increases

References		
130.1 BNF	s 1.2	
130.2 Dundee	p 210–211	
130.3 BNF	s 1.6.2	
130.4 Synopsis	p 138–141	
130.5 Rang	p 458	
131.1 Dundee	p 283–294	
131.2 Calvey	p 245	
132.1 Souhami	p 493–495	

130a) T The antimuscarinic drug atropine reduces both gastric motility and gastric emptying (130.1).
  b) T Gastric movements are reduced and the pylorus is contracted thus gastric emptying time increases (130.2).
  c) F Parasympathomimetic agents such as neostigmine increase intestinal and gastric motility. The effects are reversed by atropine (130.3).
  d) T Motility of the gastrointestinal tract is inhibited by halothane (130.4).
  e) F Metoclopramide has central antiemetic effects and exerts a local stimulant effect on gastric motility with a marked acceleration of gastric emptying but no concomitant increase in acid secretion (130.5). The use of metoclopramide in accelerating gastric emptying prior to anaesthesia should be reserved for the intravenous route of administration.

131a) F Local anaesthetic agents readily cross the placenta by passive diffusion. Their molecular size and high lipid solubility aid placental transfer (131.1).
  b) T Local anaesthetic agents are generally highly lipid soluble (131.1).
  c) T Although local anaesthetic agents can produce convulsive seizures it is recognised that lignocaine has been used in the treatment of status epilepticus (131.1, 131.2).
  d) T In both epidural and subarachnoid anaesthesia repeat doses or infusion may produce less effective and shorter acting blockade, in other words, tachyphylaxis (131.1).
  e) T The hydrochloride salt of the amide is the usual preparation (131.1).

132a) F Chronic obstructive pulmonary disease is defined as the presence of productive cough on most days for three months of the year for two or more successive years (133.1).
  b) F FEV_1 is reduced and FEV_1/FVC is low, indicating expiratory flow limitation (133.1).
  c) T Hyperinflation results in an increase in residual volume and total lung capacity (133.1).
  d) F The peak expiratory flow rate decreases (133.1).
  e) T Increased intraluminal mucus and thickening of the bronchial wall produces airway narrowing and increased airway resistance (133.1).

133 A lesion of the cauda equina may produce:
a) foot drop
b) incontinence
c) retention
d) upper motor neurone signs
e) paralysis

134 Compared to alfentanil, fentanyl has:
a) larger volume of distribution
b) shorter half-life
c) greater hepatic clearance
d) higher pKa
e) slower onset of action

135 The following statements are true:
a) the anaemia of iron deficiency is microcytic and normochromic
b) normal plasma osmolality lies between 260 and 290 mosmol/kg H_2O
c) the molecular weight of halothane is 144
d) diacetyl morphine is a prodrug
e) normal peak expiratory flow rate for an adult male is 600 ml/min

References	
133.1 Souhami	p 935
133.2 Souhami	p 877
134.1 Dundee	p 219–229
135.1 Souhami	p 1044–1045
135.2 Dunnill	p 75
135.3 Dunnill	p 7
135.4 Dundee	p 214
135.5 Dunnill	p 126

133a) T Lesions of the cauda equina produce signs of embarrassment to those nerve roots involved, namely L2–S5. Foot drop is a term used to denote lack of dorsiflexors, all of which are supplied by the sciatic nerve (root value L4–S1).

b) T Note with caution that the incontinence of urine is usually overflow in nature and hence secondary to retention. Common early symptoms are difficulty in voiding and poor stream (133.1).

c) T See (b) above (133.1).

d) F The neurological signs in the legs will be those of a lower motor neurone lesion as the lesion will by definition be below the anterior horn cell (133.2).

e) T Weakness of the leg muscles is an early sign (133.1). This may progress to frank paralysis if the lesion is left untreated for long enough.

134a) T The volume of distribution of alfentanil lies between 0.5–1 l/kg. The corresponding value for fentanyl is 3.7 l/kg (134.1).

b) F The terminal half-life of fentanyl is 3–4 h, that of alfentanil 1.5 h. It is not clear which half-life the question requires, but all the half-lives of alfentanil are shorter than those of fentanyl (134.1).

c) T Total hepatic clearance of alfentanil is lower than that for fentanyl, the extraction ratio being 0.5 (134.1).

d) T The pKa of alfentanil is 6.8 compared with 8.4 for fentanyl. This accounts for the rapid onset of alfentanil, as at plasma pH 85% will be un-ionised and thus able to penetrate neurolipid (134.1).

e) T The onset of action of alfentanil is extremely fast for the reason described above (134.1).

135a) F The classic anaemia of uncomplicated iron deficiency is hypochromic and microcytic (135.1).

b) F Normal osmolality lies between 280 and 300 mosmol/kg H_2O (135.2).

c) F The molecular weight of halothane is 197 Daltons (135.3).

d) F A prodrug requires metabolism to a secondary product before a clinical effect is seen. Diamorphine, although rapidly deacetylated to morphine, possesses its own clinical activity (135.4).

e) F Caution! The correct value is 600 litres/min (135.5).

136 Passive hyperventilation of a normal patient at twice minute volume with air results in:
a) a fall in P_{CO_2}
b) improved liberation of oxygen from oxyhaemoglobin
c) a reduction in the ratio of ionised to un-ionised calcium
d) a decrease in circulating red cells
e) an increase in cerebral oxygen tension

137 Haematemesis:
a) may be due to a Mallory-Weiss tear
b) is not associated with melaena
c) H_2-receptor antagonist drugs reduce mortality
d) may be caused by aspirin
e) can occur in chronic renal failure

138 Thiopentone 2.5% is preferred to 5% because, in accidental arterial injection:
a) the pH of 5% solution is neutral
b) the pH of 2.5% is half that of the 5% solution
c) as the 2.5% solution is less alkaline there is less vasoconstriction
d) crystals of 2.5% solution cause less damage than 5%
e) 2.5% solution does not contain sodium carbonate

References	
136.1 Synopsis	p 39–40
137.1 Souhami	p 573–575
138.1 Synopsis	p 160–165

136a) **T** P_{CO_2} may fall to half the normal value (136.1).
   b) **F** The rise in blood pH results in a reduction in liberation of oxygen and a shift of the oxygen dissociation curve to the left (136.1).
   c) **T** Ionised calcium falls and total plasma calcium rises so therefore the ratio is reduced (136.1).
   d) **F** There is an increase in circulating red cell numbers and a loss of plasma water from the circulation (136.1).
   e) **F** Cerebral blood flow is reduced with shrinkage of the brain. Cerebral oxygen tension is reduced (136.1).

137a) **T** A Mallory-Weiss tear occurs at the gastro-oesophageal junction and follows vomiting. The bleeding is usually self-limiting (137.1).
   b) **F** Depending on the speed and the volume of the bleed, fresh blood or melaena (black tarry stools) may be passed per rectum. Melaena is altered, partially digested blood (137.1).
   c) **F** Although they are now widely used, the introduction of H_2-receptor antagonist drugs has not reduced operation rates nor mortality (137.1).
   d) **T** Aspirin, alcohol, corticosteroids and non-steroidal anti-inflammatory drugs can provoke haematemesis (137.1).
   e) **T** Systemic causes include chronic renal failure and thrombocytopenia (137.1).

138a) **F** The pH of 2.5% and 5% thiopentone solutions is around 11 (138.1).
   b) **F** As explained in (a) there is no change of pH with dilution (138.1).
   c) **F** As there is no change in pH with dilution, this is not an influential factor (138.1).
   d) **F** Crystal formation from any concentration of thiopentone will cause damage. 2.5% thiopentone causes less damage than the 5% solution. It is thought to be the greater 'weight' of drug that is inevitably injected with 5% solutions that is responsible for the crystal formation. When the crystals are carried to small vessels their irritant properties cause direct noradrenaline release, vascular spasm and gangrene (138.1).
   e) **F** Thiopentone powder has 6% anhydrous sodium carbonate added to prevent formation of free acid by the action of carbon dioxide in the atmosphere. Sodium carbonate is therefore present in all solutions (138.1).

---

139 Oil/gas solubility of a volatile agent is related to:
a) potency
b) speed of onset
c) compatibility with soda lime
d) arrhythmogenicity
e) boiling point

---

140 The following are characteristics of depolarising relaxant drugs:
a) they are antagonised by anticholinesterases
b) post-tetanic potentiation occurs
c) fade occurs
d) fasciculation is seen
e) there is a train-of-four ratio of 0.75

---

141 Which of the following may be used to supplement hypotensive anaesthesia:
a) beta blockade
b) head-up tilt
c) adding halothane to the inspired mixture
d) infiltration with adrenaline-containing solutions
e) ephedrine

References	
139.1 Vickers	p 120–124
139.2 Aitkenhead	p 307
140.1 Dundee	p 298–299
141.1 Aitkenhead	p 595–602
141.2 Aitkenhead	p 265–266
141.3 Dundee	p 359–360

139a) T The correlation between oil/gas coefficient and the MAC of a volatile agent is the basis of the lipid solubility theory of the mode of action of anaesthetics (139.1). MAC is a measure of the 'potency' of a volatile agent, and the product of the oil/gas partition coefficient and the MAC of an agent is approximately constant.

b) F Blood/gas partition coefficient relates to the speed of onset. The lower the coefficient, the less soluble the agent, the more rapid the alveolar and brain tension rise and so the more rapid the induction (139.1).

c) F Trichloroethylene degenerates at the high temperatures that occur in soda lime canisters. This is a specific chemical event unrelated to solubility coefficients (139.3).

d) F There is no relationship (139.1).

e) F There is no relationship (139.1).

140a) F The main pharmacological difference between depolarising and non-depolarising relaxants is that non-depolarising agents can be antagonised by anticholinesterases such as neostigmine (140.1).

b) F Post-tetanic potentiation is a feature of non-depolarising neuromuscular blockade. It is shown as a greater response to a single stimulus than before after a burst of stimulation at 50 Hz (140.1).

c) F Fade is one of the main characteristics of a non-depolarising block (140.1).

d) T Fasciculation occurs with the onset of the effects of depolarising relaxants (140.1).

e) F In the train of four, a non-depolarising block produces a progressive reduction in the amplitude of response. In a depolarising block, all four responses are equally diminished (140.1).

141a) T Beta adrenergic blockade produces both a fall in heart rate and a reduction in myocardial contractility. These effects may be the mainstay of the induction of hypotension or an adjunct to overcome the reflex tachycardia that may occur with induction of hypotension (141.1).

b) T The decrease in pressure as the operation site is raised above the heart is of the order of 2 mmHg for every 2.5 cm. Venous pooling will also occur in dependent areas, so enhancing the effect of vasodilating agents (141.1).

c) T Halothane produces a dose-related decrease in arterial pressure by direct myocardial depression (141.1).

d) F Although infiltration of adrenaline-containing solutions may reduce bleeding at the site of the surgery, absorption can produce systemic toxicity and hypertension (141.2).

e) F Arterial pressure rises after the administration of ephedrine (141.3).

142 Vitamin B$_{12}$:
a) contains cobalt
b) is usually deficient due to inadequate dietary intake
c) may be useful in treating toxicity caused by sodium nitroprusside
d) is measured by the Schilling test
e) is found mainly in green vegetables

143 A patient requiring manipulation of a fractured long bone under anaesthesia has eaten within 1 hour of the injury. Which of the following would be reasonable to reduce the risk of aspiration during induction of anaesthesia:
a) inhalational induction in left lateral head-down position
b) insertion of a wide bore nasogastric tube
c) application of pressure to the cricoid cartilage
d) wait 6 hours before anaesthesia
e) opioid premedication

144 Inadequate depth of anaesthesia leads to:
a) lacrimation
b) regular respiration
c) mydriasis
d) hypertension
e) bradycardia

References	
142.1 Ganong	p 461–462
142.2 Souhami	p 60
142.3 Souhami	p 1046–1047
143.1 Aitkenhead	p 529–539
144.1 Aitkenhead	p 381

142a) **T** Vitamin B_{12} (cyanocobalamin) is a complex cobalt-containing vitamin that is necessary for normal erythropoiesis (142.1).
  b) **F** Deficiency states that are seen clinically are usually due to defective absorption due to lack of intrinsic factor or primary intestinal disease (142.1).
  c) **F** Dicobalt edetate can be used in the treatment of cyanide poisoning from sodium nitroprusside (142.2).
  d) **T** Urinary excretion of orally administered radioactively labelled vitamin B_{12} is measured in the Schilling test. The Schilling test is used for the diagnosis of the cause of B_{12} deficiency and full details can be found in the reference (142.3).
  e) **F** Animal products are the main source of B_{12} in the diet (142.3).

143a) **F** Inhalational induction is only recommended if there is doubt about ability to maintain or secure a patent airway (143.1).
  b) **F** Insertion of a nasogastric tube and aspiration of gastric contents is suitable for liquid gastric contents that occurs in bowel obstruction but is of little value for solid gastric contents (143.1).
  c) **T** Cricoid pressure or Sellick's manoeuvre, is part of a rapid sequence induction. Application results in the oesophagus being compressed between the cricoid cartilage and the vertebral column (143.1).
  d) **F** Fear, pain, shock and treatment with opioids after dislocation or fracture reduce gastric emptying. Time between ingestion of food and accident is a more reliable guide of starvation status. Although the 6-hour rule is normally observed this may not always be a helpful precaution (143.1).
  e) **F** See (d) above (143.1).

144a) **T** A 'light' anaesthetic may lead to awareness. Signs of awareness include restlessness, sweating, reactive pupils, irregular respiration (if breathing is spontaneous) hypertension, tachycardia and lacrimation (144.1).
  b) **F** In spontaneously breathing patients irregular respiration is a sign of lightness (144.1).
  c) **T** Mydriasis (pupillary dilatation) occurs during light anaesthesia. Reactive pupils occur during light states and may indicate awareness (144.1).
  d) **T** See (a) (144.1).
  e) **F** Tachycardia occurs (144.1).

145 Indications for elective post-operative ventilation include:
a) extreme obesity
b) gastric acid aspiration
c) severe pulmonary disease
d) sepsis
e) prolonged shock

146 In a patient with severe burns:
a) the arm represents 9% of the total body surface area
b) hyperkalaemia may follow suxamethonium
c) 50% of the fluid given after the first 24 hours should be blood
d) carboxyhaemoglobin may be present
e) tracheostomy is essential if the face is burnt

147 The oesophagus:
a) lies in the anterior mediastinum
b) ends about 20 cm from the teeth
c) is lined by columnar epithelium
d) starts at C6
e) does not enter the abdomen

References		
145.1 Aitkenhead		p 535–536
146.1 Nimmo		p 1474–1485
146.2 Mason		p 38–41
146.3 Aitkenhead		p 583–586
147.1 Gray's		p 1331–1333

145a) T Indications for continuation of ventilatory assistance post-operatively are tabulated in the reference (145.1). They include: prolonged shock or hypoperfusion, massive sepsis, severe ischaemic heart disease, extreme obesity, gastric aspiration and previously severe pulmonary disease (145.1).
b) T See (a) above (145.1).
c) T See (a) above (145.1).
d) T Common causes of massive sepsis include: faecal peritonitis, cholangitis and septicaemia (145.1).
e) T Prolonged shock or hypoperfusion state of any cause may require post-operative prophylactic ventilation (145.1).

146a) T The 'rule of nines' refers to percentage of body surface area represented by different parts of the body. The arms and head each contribute 9%, the front and back of the torso each contribute 18%, each leg contributes 18% and the genitalia contribute 1% (146.1).
b) T For the period of 20 to 60 days after injury, in the presence of muscle damage, the administration of suxamethonium may release potassium into the circulation with subsequent cardiac arrest (146.2).
c) F During the first 24 hours 50% of the fluid replacement volume should be given as colloid (e.g. human albumin solution). If the burns involve extensive full thickness areas then some of the colloid volume should include whole blood (146.2).
d) T Smoke inhalation leads to carbon monoxide poisoning. The diagnosis may be proven by testing for the presence of carboxyhaemoglobin (146.1).
e) F A tracheostomy is generally regarded as undesirable because of the increase in the risk of infection and the consequences of infection in damaged tissue surrounding the area (146.3).

147a) F The oesophagus descends through the anterior and posterior mediastina anterior to the vertebral column (147.1).
b) F The oesophagus starts 15 cm from the incisor teeth and traverses the diaphragm 40 cm from the incisor teeth (147.1).
c) F The lining is non-keratinising stratified squamous epithelium (147.1).
d) T The origin is level with the lower cricoid border and the sixth cervical vertebra (147.1).
e) F The oesophagus traverses the diaphragm at the level of the tenth thoracic vertebra and ends at the gastro-cardiac orifice (at the level of the eleventh thoracic vertebra). The section below the diaphragm is named the 'abdominal part' (147.1).

148 The clinical features of constrictive pericarditis include:
a) fourth heart sound
b) pulsus paradoxus
c) high incidence of murmurs
d) ascites
e) bounding pulse

149 With respect to the jugular venous pulse:
a) the 'a' wave is due to ventricular systole
b) the 'c' wave is caused by the bulging of the pulmonary valve during isometric contraction
c) the 'v' wave corresponds to the rise in atrial pressure before the opening of the tricuspid valve
d) cannon waves are not seen in complete heart block
e) a giant 'a' wave is not seen in complete heart block

150 The following features are true of the arterial pulse:
a) the rate of travel of pulse wave is higher in the large arteries than in the aorta
b) the pulse wave travels faster with advanced age
c) the pulse wave is accentuated in aortic incompetence
d) a water hammer pulse is seen in aortic incompetence
e) the dichrotic notch is caused by the vibrations of the pulmonary valve

References	
148.1 Souhami	p 435
149.1 Ganong	p 478
150.1 Ganong	p 478

148a) F In constrictive pericarditis heart sounds are generally faint with a loud additional third heart sound which results from the impeding of ventricular filling by the relatively rigid pericardium (148.1).

b) T Pulsus paradoxus (exaggerated diminution of pulse pressure and volume with respiration) is a clinical feature of restrictive pericarditis (148.1).

c) F The incidence of murmurs is low (148.1).

d) T Severe oedema accompanied by ascites and liver engorgement is a classical presentation (148.1).

e) F The character of the pulse in constrictive pericarditis is collapsing (148.1).

149a) F The 'a' wave is due to atrial systole (149.1).

b) F The 'c' wave is caused by the transmission of the rise in atrial pressure produced by the bulging of the underlying tricuspid valve into the atria during isometric ventricular contraction (149.1).

c) T The 'v' wave parallels the rise in atrial pressure before the tricuspid valve opens during diastole (149.1).

d) F When atrial contraction occurs against a closed tricuspid valve (a situation that occurs in atrio-ventricular dissociation) a cannon wave occurs (149.1).

e) F A giant 'a' wave is synonymous with a cannon wave (149.1).

150a) T The arterial pulse wave travels at 4 m/s in the aorta and 8 m/s in the large arteries (150.1).

b) T Due to the arterial tree becoming increasingly rigid with age the arterial pulse wave moves faster (150.1).

c) T Aortic incompetence results in a particularly strong pulse wave (150.1).

d) T The character of the pulse in aortic incompetence is collapsing or 'water hammer'. The water hammer was a 19th century toy detailed in the reference (150.1).

e) F The dichrotic notch, a small oscillation on the descent of the pulse wave is caused by the closing of the aortic valve cusps (150.1).

151 Diethyl ether:
a) is explosive
b) is associated with a high incidence of arrhythmias
c) is mainly metabolised to halogenated compounds
d) causes PONV
e) has a MAC of 19.2

152 Which of the following antiemetics are associated with extrapyramidal side effects:
a) metoclopramide
b) hyoscine
c) droperidol
d) prochlorperazine
e) cyclizine

153 Etomidate:
a) reduces intracranial pressure
b) is formulated in 35% propylene glycol
c) is excreted unchanged by the kidney
d) causes more venous sequelae than thiopentone
e) releases histamine

References		
151.1 Synopsis		p 917–918
152.1 BNF		s 4.6
152.2 BNF		s 4.2.1
153.1 Dundee		p 155–159

151a) T Diethyl ether is flammable in air at concentrations between 2% and 50%. It is explosive in oxygen between 2% and 80% (151.1).
  b) F Arrhythmias under diethyl ether anaesthesia are rare (151.1).
  c) F Diethyl ether is excreted mostly unchanged; 90% is eliminated by the lungs, with a minor metabolic route yielding alcohol, acetaldehyde and acetic acid (151.1).
  d) T PONV (post-operative nausea and vomiting) occurs in more than half the number of patients anaesthetised with diethyl ether (151.1).
  e) F The MAC of diethyl ether is 1.92 (151.1).

152a) T The incidence of extrapyramidal side effects is particularly high in children and young adults (152.1).
  b) F Hyoscine, which acts on the vomiting centre, is not associated with extrapyramidal side effects (152.1).
  c) T The association exists (152.2).
  d) T Note also that the comment on the incidence of extrapyramidal side effects in (a) applies (152.1).
  e) F Extrapyramidal side effects are not seen (152.1).

153a) T Etomidate reduces ICP and cerebral blood flow in a similar manner to thiopentone (153.1).
  b) T The commercial preparation of etomidate is a 0.2% solution in a 35% propylene glycol solvent (153.1).
  c) F Etomidate is mostly metabolised to yield inactive metabolites. Only 2% of an administered dose is excreted unchanged in the urine (153.1).
  d) T 25% of patients complain of venous irritation. In contrast, 4% of patients show thrombophlebitis after thiopentone (153.1).
  e) F Etomidate does not release 'significant' quantities of histamine. Answer at your peril. 'False' is the authors' choice (153.1).

154 A thermistor:
a) demonstrates the Seebeck effect
b) shows a linear relationship between resistance and temperature
c) has a resistance that changes with time
d) exhibits hysteresis
e) may have positive or negative temperature coefficients

155 The following cylinder pressures are correct when full:
a) oxygen 1980 psi
b) nitrous oxide 640 psi or 5×10^3 kPa
c) carbon dioxide 5×10^3 kPa
d) carbon dioxide 700 psi
e) oxygen 135 atm

156 Pyridostigmine:
a) is more potent than neostigmine
b) has a longer duration of action than neostigmine
c) has a slower onset of action than neostigmine
d) causes more arrhythmias than neostigmine
e) may be used for reversing non-depolarising muscle relaxant drugs

References	
154.1 Sykes	p 280
155.1 Ward	p 32–33
156.1 Synopsis 10e	p 273

154a) F The Seebeck effect is the generation of electromotive force at a junction of two different metals. It is employed in a thermocouple (154.1).

b) F Over the range of body temperature, resistance varies non-linearly with temperature. Electronic circuitry is employed to correct this (154.1).

c) T Thermistors show 'ageing', that is to say a change in resistance with time (154.1).

d) T Hysteresis is seen, such that the value of a given temperature during the heating cycle is less than the value during a cooling cycle (for any one temperature) (154.1).

e) T Thermistors may be manufactured to have positive or negative temperature coefficients (154.1).

155a) T This may also be expressed as 140 kg/cm^2 or 135 atm (155.1).

b) F 640 psi is correct but this equates to 4.4×10^3 kPa (155.1).

c) T Equivalent to 723 psi (155.1).

d) F See (c) above (155.1).

e) T See (a) above (155.1).

156a) F Pyridostigmine has one quarter of the potency of neostigmine (156.1).

b) T The duration of action of pyridostigmine (6 h) is longer than that of neostigmine (156.1).

c) T The onset of action of pyridostigmine is slower than that of neostigmine (156.1).

d) F Cardiac arrhythmias are said to be less common (156.1).

e) T Pyridostigmine has been particularly advocated for the reversal of non-depolarising relaxants in cases of renal failure due to its long duration of action (156.1).

157 A patient with rheumatoid arthritis may be expected to be:
a) anaemic
b) hypovolaemic
c) hypotensive
d) difficult to intubate
e) oedematous

158 Digoxin may be useful in the treatment of:
a) atrial fibrillation
b) heart failure
c) 2 to 1 heart block
d) ventricular tachycardia
e) multiple ventricular ectopics

159 Pressure:
a) relates force to area
b) relates flow to area
c) can be measured by a column of fluid
d) is measured in N/m^2
e) is the force acting per unit mass

References	
157.1 Souhami	p 985–989
157.2 Synopsis	p 407
158.1 BNF	s 2.1.1
159.1 Scurr	p 18–22

157a) T Anaemia is the commonest extra-articular feature of rheumatoid arthritis (157.1).
  b) F In a chronic disease such as rheumatoid arthritis, hypovolaemia does not occur (157.1).
  c) F Pulmonary hypertension may occur secondary to other rheumatoid pulmonary disease but systemic hypertension does not occur (157.1).
  d) T Laryngoscopy may be difficult due to flexion deformity of the cervical vertebrae and involvement of the temperomandibular joints (157.2). Great care may be needed during intubation. In 25% of rheumatoid patients requiring reconstructive joint surgery atlanto-axial dislocation is present and neck manipulation may result in vertebrobasilar insufficiency or spinal cord damage (157.1).
  e) T Recurrent oedema of the lower limbs occurs. Although this is sometimes related to joint disease there is frequently no obvious cause (157.1).

158a) T Atrial fibrillation is the main indication for the use of digoxin (158.1).
  b) T Digoxin can be useful in the treatment of mild heart failure even in patients in sinus rhythm. Diuretics and vasodilators are more effective and thus more frequently used (158.1).
  c) F Atrioventricular block is an unwanted effect of digoxin (158.1).
  d) F Ventricular tachycardia and atrial tachycardia are unwanted effects of digoxin (158.1).
  e) F Ventricular extrasystoles are an unwanted side effect of digoxin (158.1).

159a) T Pressure is a precise term and is defined as the force acting normally (perpendicularly) per unit area (159.1).
  b) F See (a) above (159.1).
  c) T A manometer is a column of fluid in a tube, for example a simple mercury barometer (159.1).
  d) T N/m^2 relates to the definition. The unit in common use is the Pascal (Pa) (159.1).
  e) F See (a) above (159.1).

160 **The following statements are true of hetastarch (Hespan):**
   a) molecular weight 30 000 Daltons
   b) potassium content 5 mmol/l
   c) sodium content 150 mmol/l
   d) anaphylaxis does not occur
   e) osmolarity 310 mosm/l

161 **Clinical features of pneumothorax include:**
   a) chest pain
   b) breathlessness
   c) productive cough
   d) dull percussion note
   e) reduced breath sounds

162 **Dextran 70:**
   a) is metabolised in the liver
   b) has a molecular weight of 40 000 Daltons
   c) is antithrombogenic
   d) is a polypeptide
   e) may be used to reduce the incidence of DVT

References	
160.1 Data Sheet	p 427
161.1 Souhami	p 435
162.1 Dundee	p 551

160a) F Although different formulations of Hetastarch may have different molecular weights, the one referred to has an average molecular weight of 450 000 Daltons (160.1).
  b) F There is no potassium in the solution (160.1).
  c) F Sodium is present at a concentration of 154 mmol/l. The commercial solution (Hespan) consists of 6 g of hetastarch, 0.9 g sodium chloride and water with sodium hydroxide added to adjust pH to 5.5 (160.1).
  d) F There is a risk of anaphylaxis with all the available plasma expanding solutions. Mild sensitivity reactions only have been reported with hetastarch which is less antigenic than gelatins (160.1).
  e) T The osmolarity of hetastarch is 310 mosm/l (160.1).

161a) T The chest pain which accompanies pneumothorax is usually lateral and radiates to the shoulder (161.1).
  b) T Breathlessness usually accompanies the development of spontaneous pneumothorax if the degree of lung collapse is large. It may not be a severe symptom in small pneumothoraces (161.1).
  c) F The characteristic cough is dry and irritating in nature (161.1).
  d) F The percussion note over the affected lung is hyper-resonant (161.1).
  e) T The breath sounds over the affected lung are reduced (161.1).

162a) T Dextran is metabolised in the liver to carbon dioxide and water (162.1).
  b) F Dextran 70 has an average molecular weight of 70 000 Daltons. Dextran 40 has an average molecular weight of 40 000 Daltons (162.1).
  c) T Dextran 70 has an antithrombogenic effect due to a reduction in platelet stickiness and a reduction in factor VIII activity (162.1).
  d) F The family of dextrans belong to the polysaccharides (162.1).
  e) T There is still controversy surrounding the effectiveness of dextran 70 as a prophylactic against DVT. The benefit cannot be considered unequivocal but reports are generally 'encouraging' (162.1).

163 The brisk loss of 500 ml of blood in a healthy adult will cause:
a) a fall in systolic blood pressure
b) tachycardia
c) postural hypotension
d) a fall in diastolic blood pressure
e) thirst

164 Anaphylaxis:
a) can be avoided by prophylactic chlorpheniramine
b) occurs in 2% of patients given polygelatine
c) may cause diarrhoea
d) may recover spontaneously
e) may result in asystole

165 The following may be expected after a laparotomy in a 70-year-old man:
a) Pa_{O_2} of 8 kPa
b) an increase in FRC
c) atelectasis
d) an increase in closing volume
e) increased compliance

References	
163.1 Synopsis	p 793
163.2 Synopsis 10e	p 743
164.1 Aitkenhead	p 418–419
165.1 Aitkenhead	p 430–431

163a) F The signs and symptoms of up to 15% blood loss (750 ml) are: normal blood pressure, tachycardia and postural hypotension (163.1). 500 ml is a 10% blood loss (163.2).
  b) T See (a) above (163.1, 163.2).
  c) T Although compensation is adequate, it may not be able to cope with sudden changes in position (163.1).
  d) F There is no change in blood pressure (163.1, 163.2).
  e) F Thirst is a symptom that develops after 15–30% blood loss (163.1).

164a) F For a known drug sensitivity prophylaxis with antihistamines or steroids has been tried but has not been noted to be successful (164.1).
  b) F Incidence varies depending on source but 0.068% is quoted most commonly (164.1).
  c) T Gastrointestinal manifestations include cramping abdominal pains, nausea, vomiting and diarrhoea (164.1). Usually the anaesthetist is concerned with the more life-threatening features.
  d) T Spontaneous recovery may occur in many reactions but severe untreated reactions are fatal (164.1).
  e) T Asystole or VF may occur. Profound vasodilatation may result in absent pulses without cardiac arrest (164.1).

165a) T Even if the patient's lungs were normal pre-operatively, impaired oxygenation with a fall in Pao_2 of up to 4 kPa will occur for at least 48 hours (165.1).
  b) F The functional residual capacity (FRC) decreases soon after induction of anaesthesia and may remain reduced for 4–5 days after upper abdominal surgery (165.1).
  c) T A reduction in FRC may lead to the closing capacity approaching the tidal breathing range. This results in closure of airways during normal breathing and gas trapping. When the trapped gas is absorbed atelectasis occurs (165.1).
  d) T Closing volume increases and tidal volume decreases (165.1).
  e) F Compliance will decrease as a result of atelectasis (165.1).

166 The following associations exist:
a) lithotomy position and asymmetrical lung ventilation
b) lithotomy position and backache
c) Trendelenberg position and abdominal compression
d) prone position and corneal damage
e) lateral position and asymmetrical lung ventilation

167 The following may precipitate angina:
a) aortic stenosis
b) anaemia
c) bradycardia
d) hypertension
e) aortic regurgitation

168 Compared with plasma, CSF contains:
a) less glucose
b) more sodium
c) more urea
d) less hydrogen ions
e) less osmotically active particles

References	
166.1 Aitkenhead	p 351–352
167.1 Davidson's	p 304–305
168.1 Dunnill	p 85

166a) F Lithotomy position is not associated with unequal ventilation between the two lungs which is a feature of lateral patient positions (166.1).
b) T There is an incidence of backache after positioning in lithotomy which may be reduced if care is taken to elevate both legs simultaneously. This avoids pelvic asymmetry and sacro-iliac strain (166.1).
c) T Trendelenburg position produces a degree of abdominal compression due to the upward pressure on the diaphragm from the abdominal contents. Generally, abdominal compression is associated with prone positions (166.1).
d) T Care must be taken to cover the eyes when positioning patients prone. If corneas are left exposed ulceration may result (along with legal action!) (166.1).
e) T See (a) above (166.1).

167a) T Angina will be precipitated by any condition that increases myocardial oxygen requirement (or reduces supply). Aortic stenosis is a condition which increases work due to raised afterload (167.1).
b) T A well documented precipitator of angina, anaemia increases preload in a hyperdynamic circulation (167.1).
c) F Bradycardia maximises the time available for coronary artery perfusion during diastole. In contrast, tachycardia may precipitate angina due to reduced diastolic flow (167.1).
d) T Hypertension presents an increased afterload and thus increases myocardial workload (167.1).
e) T Aortic regurgitation reduces diastolic coronary flow (167.1).

168a) T CSF glucose concentration is normally about 1 mmol/l less than the plasma value (168.1).
b) F The sodium concentration in CSF is around 140 mmol/l. It is not higher than the plasma value (168.1).
c) F The urea level in CSF approximates to that in plasma (168.1).
d) F CSF has a slightly lower pH range than plasma (7.30–7.35). This implies more hydrogen ions (168.1).
e) F The osmolality of CSF is 306 mosm/kg. The corresponding blood value is 280–300 mosm/kg (168.1).

169 The following are features of TUR syndrome:
a) confusion
b) hypernatraemia
c) haemolysis
d) pulmonary oedema
e) hypotension

170 Muscle pains after suxamethonium may be prevented by:
a) self-taming
b) lignocaine
c) dantrolene
d) diazepam
e) tubocurarine

171 Malignant hyperthermia:
a) is inherited as Mendelian dominant
b) may be triggered by halothane
c) may be triggered by nitrous oxide
d) has a high mortality
e) results in acidosis

References		
169.1 Aitkenhead		p 424
169.2 Aitkenhead		p 489
169.3 Synopsis		p 595–6
170.1 Synopsis		p 209–210
171.1 Dundee		p 567–568

169a) T Hypo-osmolar (TUR) syndrome is a potent cause of confusion often leading to convulsions and coma following trans-urethral resection of the prostate gland (TURP) (169.1).

b) F Hyponatraemia occurs. A serum sodium of less than 120 mmol/l is considered to be diagnostic of the syndrome (169.2).

c) T Intraoperative haemolysis occurs and may cause renal damage later (169.2).

d) T Water absorption and hyponatraemia may lead to cerebral or pulmonary oedema, raised blood pressure, acute left ventricular failure and cardiac arrest (169.3).

e) F Water intoxication may lead to bradycardia and a rise in both systolic and diastolic arterial pressures (169.3). The first sign during general anaesthesia may be widening of the QRS complex and T wave inversion caused by hyponatraemia (169.3).

170a) T Self-taming is the injection of 10 mg of suxamethonium 1 minute before induction of anaesthesia. This may be unpleasant for the patient (170.1).

b) T Intravenous lignocaine (2-6 mg/kg) following thiopentone and 3 min. before the suxamethonium prevents myalgia, prolongs apnoea, and restricts the increase in serum potassium and calcium (170.1).

c) T A single oral dose of 100-150 mg dantrolene at least 2 hours pre-operatively reduces the incidence of myalgia (170.1).

d) T 10 mg of diazepam before induction reduces myalgia (170.1).

e) T A small dose of any non-depolarising drug will prevent (or reduce) the myalgia from suxamethonium (170.1).

171a) F Although originally this was thought to be the mode of inheritance, it is now known that several genes are involved, leading to different degrees of susceptibility (171.1).

b) T All vapours have been implicated but halothane is the most well known example of a volatile trigger agent (171.1).

c) F Nitrous oxide (if administered from uncorrupt equipment) is safe to use in susceptible patients (171.1).

d) T The mortality after the acute event is around 60% (171.1).

e) T Respiratory and metabolic acidoses with hyperkalaemia are usual (171.1).

172 Air embolism:
a) may be accompanied by paradoxical embolism
b) increases CVP
c) causes an early fall in oxygen saturation
d) decreases PAWP
e) causes a reduction in end tidal CO_2 tension

173 Symptoms and signs of thyrotoxicosis include:
a) papilloedema
b) gruff voice
c) cold intolerance
d) diplopia
e) dysphagia

174 With respect to the metabolism of suxamethonium:
a) plasma cholinesterase deficiency can be acquired in pregnancy
b) atypical cholinesterase shows Mendelian dominant inheritance
c) dibucaine number of 80 is normal
d) cholinesterase is found in the red cells
e) normal cholinesterase level is 50 units/ml

References
172.1 Mason   p 443–445
173.1 Souhami   p 694–699
174.1 Synopsis   p 205–208

172a) T Paradoxical embolus occurs when air enters the left side of the heart and can thence cause an embolus in the arterial system. It can occur in the presence of a patent foramen ovale (20%–35% of patients at post mortem) and may occur in 10% of patients undergoing operations predisposing to entry of air into the venous system (172.1).
b) T Late signs of a significant air embolus include: a rise in CVP, a rise in pulmonary arterial wedge pressure (PAWP), hypotension, arrhythmias and a fall in oxygen saturation (172.1).
c) F A fall in oxygen saturation is a late sign (172.1).
d) F PAWP increases. See (b) above (172.1).
e) T A fall in end tidal carbon dioxide tension is an early sign (172.1).

173a) T Papilloedema is a local effect in Grave's disease due to raised orbital pressure (173.1).
b) F A gruff voice is a sign of myxoedema (173.1).
c) F Cold intolerance is a symptom of myxoedema (173.1).
d) T Diplopia is a symptom of thyrotoxicosis (173.1).
e) T Dysphagia occurs as a result of compression of the oesophagus (173.1).

174a) T Pregnancy is a cause of acquired cholinesterase deficiency and can reveal an otherwise seemingly normal heterozygous state (174.1).
b) F The inheritance is Mendelian recessive (174.1).
c) T Normal dibucaine number (DN) ranges from 75 to 85 (174.1).
d) F Plasma cholinesterase is found in: plasma, liver, brain, kidneys and pancreas (174.1).
e) F Normal plasma cholinesterase levels are about 80 units/ml (174.1).

175 Spinal opioids are associated with:
a) nausea and vomiting
b) respiratory depression
c) pruritus
d) shivering
e) retention of urine

176 Exchanging nitrogen in the atmosphere for helium will result in:
a) increased density
b) easier breathing in patients with upper airway obstruction
c) hypnosis
d) higher specific gravity
e) increased flammability

177 The following are SI base units:
a) degree Celsius
b) candela
c) metre per second
d) ampere
e) mole

References	
175.1 Review 9	p 80–95
176.1 Synopsis 10e	p 202–203
177.1 Scurr	p 8–9

175a) T The incidence of nausea and vomiting after intrathecal opioids is high. It is somewhat lower if the epidural route is used but remains a clinical problem (175.1).

b) T Respiratory depression may occur after the intrathecal administration of opioid agents and this may be delayed in onset. Naloxone may be used to reverse the effect (175.1).

c) T Pruritus is common after intrathecal opioids, particularly with morphine, diamorphine and fentanyl (incidence 50%). It is less common (10%) when the epidural route is used (175.1).

d) F Shivering is associated with the use of local anaesthetic agents, not opioids (175.1).

e) T The precise incidence is not known but the association exists (175.1).

176a) F Helium is an inert gas of low density. Replacing nitrogen in the atmosphere with helium lowers the specific gravity. Density is thus reduced (176.1).

b) T The reduction in density will increase flow in turbulent flow situations (such as upper airway obstruction). Helium is used in such situations clinically in a mixture of helium/oxygen (176.1).

c) F Helium is an inert gas without hypnotic effects (176.1).

d) F The specific gravity of an 80% helium/20% oxygen mixture is 341, that of air 1000 (176.1).

e) F Helium is inert (176.1).

177a) F SI base units are single units of quantity which carry official and precise definitions. The SI base unit of temperature is the Kelvin, not degree Celsius. It is defined as 1/273.16 of the thermodynamic triple point of water (177.1).

b) T The candela is the SI base unit of luminosity (177.1).

c) F Metre per second is a unit of speed and rather than being a base unit it is a compound unit (177.1).

d) T The ampere is the SI base unit of current. It is defined as that constant current which, if maintained in two straight parallel conductors of infinite length, of negligible cross-sectional area, one metre apart in a vacuum, would produce a force of 2×10^{-7} Newtons per metre of length (177.1).

e) T A mole is an SI base unit. It is that amount of a substance which contains the same number of elementary particles as atoms in 0.012 kg of carbon[12] (177.1).

178 Naloxone reverses respiratory depression secondary to:
a) pentazocine
b) nalbuphine
c) buprenorphine
d) diazepam
e) fentanyl

179 Flumazenil:
a) will reverse the sedative effects of diazepam
b) can precipitate convulsions
c) will reverse the sedative effects of fentanyl
d) will reverse the sedative effects of halothane
e) can cause ventricular arrhythmias

180 Insulin increases:
a) protein catabolism
b) gluconeogenesis
c) amino acid entry into cells
d) serum potassium
e) uptake of glucose by fat cells

References	
178.1 Dundee	p 221–225
179.1 BNF	s 15.1.7
179.2 Dundee	p 190–191
180.1 Guyton	p 855–860

178a) T Naloxone reverses the respiratory depression caused by opioid receptor agonists (178.1).
b) T See (a) (178.1).
c) F No satisfactory antagonist to respiratory depression caused by buprenorphine exists (178.1). Naloxone may be partially effective, but due to high binding affinity of buprenorphine to receptors it is unlikely to fully reverse the effects of buprenorphine.
d) F Diazepam is not an opioid agonist (178.1).
e) T See (a) (178.1).

179a) T Flumazenil reverses the sedative effects of benzodiazepines (179.1).
b) T Convulsions are a rare side effect. The drug should not be used in epileptic patients on long term benzodiazepines (179.1).
c) F Fentanyl is not a benzodiazepine (179.1).
d) T Flumazenil has been found to hasten recovery from halothane anaesthesia although the mechanism is unknown (179.2).
e) T Ventricular arrhythmias have been recorded (179.2).

180a) F Insulin promotes protein anabolism (180.1).
b) F Gluconeogenesis is inhibited. Gluconeogenesis is the formation of carbohydrates from proteins and fats (180.1).
c) T Insulin promotes active transport of amino acids into the cells (180.1).
d) F The activity of the sodium-potassium ATPase of the sodium-potassium pump is increased. Cellular uptake of potassium increases and the plasma level thus falls (180.1).
e) T Glucose transport through the fat cell membrane is facilitated by insulin (180.1).

181 Mivacurium:
a) releases histamine
b) increases mean arterial pressure
c) is metabolised by cholinesterase
d) is not eliminated in urine
e) is long acting

182 The following reduce cerebral blood flow:
a) Pa_{CO_2} 8–11 kPa
b) thiopentone
c) ketamine
d) halothane
e) hypoxic mixtures

183 Alcuronium:
a) does not release histamine
b) causes tachycardia
c) is poorly protein bound
d) causes hypotension
e) is excreted in the urine

References	
181.1 Synopsis	p 202
182.1 Synopsis	p 492–500
183.1 Dundee	p 304–305

181a) T Mivacurium appears not to be a potent liberator of histamine. More prolonged usage is necessary to confirm this (181.1).
b) F Heart rate and arterial pressure are lowered (181.1).
c) T Mivacurium is hydrolysed by plasma cholinesterase (181.1).
d) F The products of hydrolysis are excreted in both bile and urine (181.1).
e) F Mivacurium has a short duration of action which approximates to twice that of suxamethonium (181.1).

182a) F Hypercapnia of such a degree will increase cerebral blood flow by a factor of 100% (182.1).
b) T Thiopentone, methohexitone, diazepam, droperidol and fentanyl reduce cerebral blood flow (182.1).
c) F Ketamine may have little effect on cerebral blood flow in low doses but cerebral vasodilation is seen at higher doses (182.1).
d) F All the inhalational agents increase cerebral blood flow (182.1).
e) F Hypoxic mixtures raise cerebral blood flow. Inspired oxygen concentrations around 10% increase cerebral blood flow by 30% or so (182.1).

183a) T Alcuronium causes release of histamine to a lesser extent than does curare (183.1).
b) T Tachycardia is generally seen (183.1).
c) F Alcuronium is strongly bound to albumin (183.1).
d) T The hypotensive effect is dose-dependent and similar in severity to curare (183.1).
e) T 80–85% of a dose of alcuronium is recoverable from the urine. The remainder is excreted in bile and faeces (183.1).

184 The Boyle's anaesthetic machine:
a) was invented by the same person responsible for the gas law
b) cannot be used for neonates
c) includes a plenum vaporiser
d) is a demand machine
e) back bar pressure relief valve protects patients from barotrauma

185 Recognised complications of laryngoscopy are:
a) sublingual haematoma
b) arytenoid dislocation
c) epistaxis
d) epiglottic haematoma
e) hypotension

186 Dextran 70:
a) has a lower molecular weight than gelatine
b) should not be used in patients with renal impairment
c) can only be used with saline
d) may cause hypotension
e) interferes with cross-matching

References	
184.1 Ward	p 94–112
185.1 Nimmo	p 451–452
186.1 Aitkenhead	p 136–137

184a) F The two were different people. For a full description see question 70(d).
  b) F Breathing circuits and ventilators are specific to neonatal anaesthesia but a Boyle's machine can be used to supply the gas (184.1).
  c) F There are connections on the back bar for vaporisers but these are not specifically included as part of the Boyle's machine (184.1).
  d) F The Boyle's machine supplies a continuous flow of anaesthetic gases (184.1).
  e) F The back bar pressure relief valve opens the back bar to the atmosphere at 30–40 kPa. Its purpose is to protect the machine, not the patient (184.1).

185a) T Hazards of laryngoscopy include: damage to lips, teeth, dental prostheses, gingivae, tongue and epiglottis. Another complication can be arytenoid dislocation (185.1).
  b) T See (a) (185.1).
  c) F Epistaxis may be a complication of nasal intubation but the concept of nasal damage during laryngoscopy is difficult to comprehend (185.1).
  d) T See (a). Damage may occur in any part of the larynx that the laryngoscope blade contacts (185.1).
  e) F Laryngoscopy may lead to sympatho-adrenal stimulation with resultant hypertension (185.1).

186a) F The 70 of dextran 70 refers to the molecular weight of 70 000 Daltons. The molecular weight of the gelatins (Haemaccel® or Gelofusine®) is 30 000–35 000 Daltons (186.1).
  b) T Dextrans should not be used in patients with renal impairment, severe congestive cardiac failure or thrombocytopaenia (186.1).
  c) F Dextran 70 is supplied as a 6% solution in either 5% dextrose or 0.9% saline (186.1).
  d) T Acute anaphylactic reactions occur resulting in erythema, bronchospasm, urticaria and hypertension (186.1).
  e) T Dextrans can cause difficulty in grouping and cross-matching by rouleaux formation of the red cells. They may also interfere with haemostatic mechanisms (186.1).

187 Droperidol has the following associations:
   a) dystonic reactions
   b) vasodilatation
   c) emesis
   d) sedation
   e) alpha blockade

---

188 Doxapram:
   a) is an analeptic drug
   b) has a wide therapeutic ratio
   c) may cause fits
   d) acts on peripheral chemoreceptors
   e) stimulates the cortex more than respiration

---

189 Clinical features of chronic bronchitis include:
   a) clubbing
   b) expiratory wheeze
   c) weight gain
   d) cor pulmonale
   e) less dyspnoea in the early morning

References	
187.1 Dundee	p 246–247
188.1 Dundee	p 474
189.1 Souhami	p 494–495

187a) **T** The principal dystonic reaction which is encountered is oculogyric crisis. This may also occur after administration of haloperidol (187.1).
  b) **T** The effect of droperidol on the peripheral circulation is one of vasodilatation secondary to alpha blockade (187.1).
  c) **F** In clinical doses droperidol is an antiemetic of high efficacy (187.1).
  d) **T** Sedation and drowsiness, accompanied by dissociation, follow the administration of droperidol in clinical doses (187.1).
  e) **T** Droperidol is an alpha blocking drug (187.1).

188a) **T** Doxapram is an analeptic agent, that is to say it stimulates respiration and causes general CNS excitation (188.1).
  b) **F** Doxapram has a wider therapeutic ratio than most other analeptic drugs, but nevertheless the therapeutic ratio of doxapram is not wide (188.1).
  c) **T** The side effects of all the respiratory stimulants are similar and include hypertension and convulsions (188.1).
  d) **T** Doxapram has a selective effect on peripheral chemoreceptors in the carotid sinus (188.1).
  e) **F** Doxapram stimulates the respiratory centre more than the cerebral cortex (188.1).

189a) **T** Clubbing is a frequent clinical sign of chronic bronchitis (189.1).
  b) **T** The early signs of chronic bronchitis may be minimal but one of the earliest signs is scattered expiratory wheeze (189.1).
  c) **F** In general, weight loss is seen and this is marked in mixed pulmonary disease when emphysema is prominent. In cor pulmonale when oedema develops there may be weight gain (189.1).
  d) **T** Cor pulmonale is a late development which carries a poor prognosis (189.1).
  e) **F** Characteristically, breathing is most difficult in the early morning due to the accumulation of secretions overnight (189.1).

190 Alpha-1 antitrypsin deficiency:
    a) is more common in men
    b) is related to localised emphysema
    c) leads to radiological change in the lung apices
    d) is associated with dextrocardia
    e) is associated with clubbing

191 Sympathetic stimulation is caused by:
    a) hypoxia
    b) hypercarbia
    c) hypoglycaemia
    d) acidosis
    e) exercise

192 Adverse effects of oxygen therapy include:
    a) 'raptures of the deep'
    b) retinitis pigmentosa
    c) diminished surfactant activity
    d) fire risk
    e) chronic poisoning when concentrations of 50% are inspired

References	
190.1 Souhami	p 494–495
190.2 Souhami	p 482
190.3 Souhami	p 459
191.1 Guyton	p 201–202
191.2 Ganong	p 323
191.3 Guyton	p 235
192.1 Nunn	p 327
192.2 Synopsis	p 820–821
192.3 Ward	p 332

190a) F Alpha-1 antitrypsin deficiency is a genetic disorder equally common in men and women with an overall incidence of 1 in 5000 people (190.1).

b) T Alpha-1 antitrypsin deficiency causes emphysema which is panlobular and predominantly basal (190.1).

c) F X-ray changes are predominantly basal (190.1).

d) F Do not get confused with Kartagener's syndrome, which is a combination of dextrocardia, mucociliary dysfunction and bronchiectasis. Kartagener is a Swiss physician (190.2).

e) T Any chronic pulmonary condition (which includes alpha-1 antitrypsin deficiency) may lead to the clinical sign of finger and toe clubbing (190.3).

191a) T Hypoxia will result in a rise in sympathetic activity mediated via the chemoreceptors and via ischaemic cells in the vasomotor centre (191.1).

b) T An excess of carbon dioxide will result in stimulation of the sympathetic nervous system via the chemoreceptors (191.1).

c) T Hypoglycaemia increases secretion of five counter-regulatory hormones: adrenalin, noradrenaline, glucagon, growth hormone and cortisol (191.2).

d) T Chemoreceptor cells are sensitive to a hydrogen ion excess and the sympathetic nervous system will be stimulated as a result (191.1).

e) T There is a mass sympathetic discharge on exercise (191.3).

192a) F 'Raptures of the deep' or nitrogen narcosis, occurs as a result of breathing air under pressure. Nitrogen at a pressure of 30 atmospheres can cause full surgical anaesthesia (192.1).

b) F Be careful here. High partial pressures of oxygen can cause retrolental fibroplasia. Retrolental fibroplasia is the formation of a fibrovascular membrane posterior to the lens in the eyes of premature babies exposed to high concentrations of oxygen (192.2). Retinitis pigmentosa is hereditary and unconnected.

c) T Surfactant production is decreased (192.2).

d) T For a fire to occur in the presence of high pressure or high concentrations of oxygen there must be combustible material and a source of ignition (192.3).

e) F Chronic poisoning occurs in concentrations of over 60% at atmospheric pressure for prolonged periods (192.2).

193 The following equations are correct:

a) $\dot{Q} = \dfrac{\pi P d^2}{128 \eta l}$

b) $P = 2T/r$

c) $V = IR$

d) EMF (millivolts) $= \pm 61 \log \dfrac{\text{conc. inside}}{\text{conc. outside}}$

e) $\dfrac{VD_{anat}}{V_T} = 1 - \dfrac{\text{mixed expired } P_{CO_2}}{\text{alveolar (end-tidal) } P_{CO_2}}$

194 In Guillain-Barré syndrome:

a) maximum weakness occurs 7 days after the start of illness
b) first symptoms are motor weakness
c) symptoms respond to steroids
d) recovery may be complete
e) CSF protein is elevated

195 The causes of papilloedema include:

a) optic neuritis
b) Guillain-Barré syndrome
c) subarachnoid haemorrhage
d) polycythaemia rubra vera
e) disseminated intravascular coagulation

References

193.1	Parbrook	p 17
193.2	Ganong	p 540
193.3	Parbrook	p 182–183
193.4	Guyton	p 51
193.5	Synopsis	p 34
194.1	Souhami	p 941
195.1	Souhami	p 865

193a) F This is an incorrect representation of the Hagen-Poiseuille equation. The diameter, d, should be to the power 4 (193.1).
   b) T This is the correct form of the law of Laplace (193.2).
   c) T Ohm's law (193.3).
   d) T This is the Nernst equation (193.4).
   e) T This represents correctly the Bohr equation for the determination of dead space (193.5).

194a) F Maximum weakness is usually found between 10 and 14 days after the onset of neuropathy (194.1).
   b) F The first symptoms are usually sensory not motor (194.1).
   c) F There is no evidence that steroids improve the outcome in GBS (194.1).
   d) T Many patients make a complete recovery. Plasmapheresis may speed recovery (194.1). Evidence is contradictory.
   e) T The CSF is under normal pressure with a lymphocytosis and usually the protein level is markedly elevated (194.1).

195a) T Papilloedema may result from a wide variety of pathologies. The major groups of which are: raised intracranial pressure, venous obstruction, optic neuritis, retinal artery occlusion, optic nerve tumours, blood diseases, poisons and elevated CSF protein. All the completions to this stem are therefore correct (195.1).
   b) T
   c) T
   d) T
   e) T

196 The oxygen-haemoglobin dissociation curve shifts to the left in:
a) the pulmonary capillaries
b) the foetus
c) hypothermia
d) acidosis
e) stored blood

197 Carbon dioxide is carried in the blood:
a) mainly as bicarbonate
b) mainly as carbamino compounds
c) preferentially by oxyhaemoglobin
d) mainly in solution
e) mainly combined with haemoglobin

198 The following values are correct for isoflurane:
a) boiling point 60°C
b) MAC 1.5 vol%
c) SVP 243 mmHg
d) blood/gas solubility coefficient 1.4
e) molecular weight 185 Daltons

References	
196.1 Guyton	p 438–439
197.1 Guyton	p 440–441
198.1 Dunnill	p 7

196a) T As blood passes through the pulmonary capillaries, carbon dioxide diffuses from it, reducing the carbonic acid content and decreasing hydrogen ion concentration. These effects shift the oxygen-haemoglobin dissociation curve to the left and upwards. This is the Bohr effect (196.1).
  b) T Foetal haemoglobin produces a shift of the curve to the left, a feature which is important for transport of oxygen in the foetus (196.1).
  c) T A reduction in temperature results in a shift to the left (196.1).
  d) F Acidosis, or an increase in hydrogen ions, results in a shift to the right (196.1).
  e) T Stored blood has reduced levels of 2,3-diphosphoglycerate (2,3-DPG). As levels fall the curve moves to the left (196.1).

197a) T Approximately 70% of CO_2 carriage in the blood is as bicarbonate (197.1).
  b) F The majority is bicarbonate, only 7% or so of carbon dioxide is carried as carbamino compounds (197.1).
  c) F The combination of oxygen with haemoglobin forms a more highly acidic haemoglobin which has less tendency to combine with carbon dioxide (197.1).
  d) F The amount of carbon dioxide carried in solution is small and represents about 0.3 ml/100ml (197.1).
  e) F Approximately 30% is carried in combination with haemoglobin (197.1).

198a) F The boiling point of isoflurane is 49°C (198.1).
  b) F The MAC value for isoflurane is 1.2 vol% (198.1).
  c) F The SVP of isoflurane at 20°C is 250 mmHg. 243 mmHg is the value for halothane (198.1).
  d) T Correct (198.1).
  e) T To be strictly accurate the molecular weight of isoflurane (and its structural isomer enflurane) is 184.5 Daltons (198.1).

199 Muscles of inspiration include:
a) external intercostals
b) diaphragm
c) internal intercostals
d) rectus abdominus
e) latissimus dorsi

200 Phenoperidine:
a) is related to fentanyl
b) is less potent than pethidine
c) causes respiratory depression
d) is excreted renally
e) is metabolised to norpethidine

201 Clinical features of sickle cell anaemia include:
a) priapism
b) retinal detachment
c) consolidation
d) painless fever
e) symptom-free first year of life

References	
199.1 Ganong	p 604–605
200.1 Dundee	p 216–217
201.1 Souhami	p 1054

199a) T Although the diaphragm is the most important muscle of inspiration the external intercostal muscles have a large role (199.1).
 b) T See (a) above (199.1).
 c) F The internal intercostal muscles are muscles of expiration (199.1).
 d) F The rectus abdominus aids expiration by pulling the rib cage down and in and by increasing intra-abdominal pressure which pushes up the diaphragm (199.1).
 e) F Latissimus dorsi has no role in the mechanics of respiration.

200a) T Phenoperidine is a derivative of norpethidine which is closely related to fentanyl (200.1).
 b) F Phenoperidine is 50 times more potent than pethidine (200.1).
 c) T In common with all opioid agents (200.1).
 d) T Half of a dose is excreted in the urine, the remainder being subject to biotransformation in the liver (200.1).
 e) T One of the products of the hepatic metabolism is norpethidine (200.1).

201a) T Priapism occurs due to sickling in the corpus cavernosa (201.1).
 b) T There is a high risk of vitreous haemorrhage and retinal detachment (201.1).
 c) T Acute pulmonary infections are common. Lung changes may progress rapidly to widespread consolidation (201.1).
 d) F Fever is accompanied by severe pain requiring opioid drugs in acute episodes of sickling (201.1).
 e) F The first six months of life are usually symptom free, after which vaso-occlusive crises begin (201.1).

202 Difficulty in intubation will be increased by:
a) increase in posterior depth of the mandible
b) increased alveolar–mental distance
c) receding incisors
d) temporomandibular joint fibrosis
e) increased distance from the C1 spinous process to the occiput

203 Face masks can be cleaned using the following:
a) 5% phenol
b) formaldehyde
c) domestic dishwasher
d) lukewarm water
e) 0.1% chlorhexidine

204 Methods of sterilisation include:
a) steam at 73°C for 2 h
b) infrared light
c) gamma rays
d) hexachlorophene
e) gluteraldehyde

References	
202.1 Aitkenhead	p 408–409
203.1 Synopsis 10e	p 831–833
204.1 Synopsis 10e	p 831–833

202a) T There are eight identified anatomical features associated with difficult intubation. An increased posterior depth of the mandible hinders displacement of the mandible during intubation (202.1).
b) T An increased alveolar–mental distance means that the mandible needs to be opened widely for laryngoscopy (202.1).
c) F Protruding incisors with a relative overgrowth of the premaxilla increases the difficulty of intubation (202.1).
d) T Poor mobility of the mandible occurs with temporomandibular joint fibrosis (202.1).
e) F Decreased distance between the occiput and the spinous process of C1 is an X-ray finding that indicates possible difficult intubation. A short muscular neck is a clinical indication (202.1).

203a) F Although 1–5% phenol is used to clean surfaces and apparatus, it must not be allowed to contact patients (203.1).
b) F Formaldehyde persists after long periods of airing and may harm the skin (203.1).
c) T A domestic dishwasher that provides temperatures above 70°C using a commercial chlorine-containing detergent is adequate for killing most pathogenic organisms encountered in anaesthesia (203.1).
d) F Thorough washing in soap and water, then soaked in water between 60 and 70°C followed by rinsing in tap water of the same temperature is suitable (203.1).
e) T Soaking in 0.1% chlorhexidine for 20 min is also a suitable method for cleaning endotracheal tubes (203.1).

204a) T Usually superheated steam (high temperature steam under pressure) is used for speed, but sterilisation can be carried out at 73°C and 290 mmHg pressure for 2 h (204.1).
b) F Ultraviolet light has been used by submitting the whole operation area to the light but the staff have to be protected against sun burn! Infrared light is used for its heating properties (204.1).
c) T A lethal dose of gamma rays for bacteria is 2.5 megarads. This form of sterilisation is carried out by many manufacturers of disposable equipment (204.1).
d) T Hexachlorophene 50–70% does not lose its antiseptic properties in the presence of soap (204.1).
e) T Activated glutaraldehyde 2% (Cidex®) will kill bacteria in 15 min and spores in 3 h (204.1).

---

205 With respect to gentamicin:
a) ototoxicity is less than with amikacin
b) deafness is a potential problem
c) depolarising neuromuscular blockade may occur
d) renal damage is irreversible
e) indications include infection with *Pseudomonas aeruginosa*

---

206 The knee-jerk reflex is:
a) polysynaptic
b) initiated by receptors in the patella
c) initiated by receptors in the quadriceps
d) a response to muscle spindle stimulation
e) absent in cord transection

---

207 High serum conjugated bilirubin is found in:
a) Gilbert's syndrome
b) carcinoma of head of pancreas
c) renal failure
d) intravascular haemolysis
e) viral hepatitis

References

205.1 Dundee	p 487–488
206.1 Ganong	p 115–116
206.2 Ganong	p 192–193
207.1 Zilva	p 299
207.2 Zilva	p 290–294

205a) F Gentamicin is considerably more ototoxic than either amikacin or kanamycin (205.1).
b) T Deafness is a recognised complication of therapy with any amino-glycoside antibiotic (205.1).
c) F The action of non-depolarising blocking drugs may be potentiated (205.1).
d) F Renal damage is usually reversible and reverts after cessation of therapy (205.1).
e) T Gentamicin is recommended as a first-line agent, mainly on the grounds of cost (205.1).

206a) F The knee-jerk reflex is a good example of a monosynaptic reflex (206.1).
b) F The initiation of the knee-jerk reflex occurs when stretch receptors in the quadriceps femoris muscle are stimulated (206.1).
c) T See (b) above (206.1).
d) T The organ sensing the stretch of the muscle is the muscle spindle (206.1).
e) F Spinal reflexes are preserved in cord transection (206.2).

207a) F Gilbert's syndrome (disease) is characterised by elevated plasma bilirubin of the unconjugated type. It is a benign and familial condition (207.1).
b) T Obstruction to the outflow of bile leads to elevated levels of conjugated bilirubin. Note that most hepatic conditions will cause a rise in both conjugated and unconjugated bilirubin (207.2).
c) F Conjugated bilirubin is highly water soluble and is excreted readily even in states of poor renal function (207.2).
d) T Haemolysis is a situation of an increased load presenting to the liver. There is no bar to the conjugation of bilirubin (207.2).
e) T Both conjugated and unconjugated fractions of bilirubin are elevated (207.1).

208 The following statements apply to the Valsalva manoeuvre:
a) initially arterial pressure rises
b) heart rate is unchanged
c) peripheral resistance falls
d) it is followed by an increase in arterial pressure
e) it is defined as a forced expiration against a closed glottis

209 Sellick's manoeuvre:
a) is the same as cricoid pressure
b) is performed by compressing the trachea with the cricoid cartilage
c) does not distort the glottis
d) may be used to prevent vomiting
e) prevents regurgitation

210 Tumours may cause:
a) hypercalcaemia
b) hyponatraemia
c) hypokalaemia
d) hyperthyroidism
e) hypoglycaemia

References	
208.1 Ganong	p 558–559
209.1 Synopsis	p 275
210.1 Zilva	p 419

208a) T Initially at the onset of straining arterial pressure rises as intrathoracic pressure is added to that in the aorta (208.1).
  b) F Tachycardia is seen firstly due to baroreceptor stimulation. Bradycardia is seen at the end of the manoeuvre when a reflex drop in heart rate accompanies the hypertension which follows the ejection of cardiac output into a circulation which has become vasoconstricted (208.1).
  c) F Decreased pulse pressure at the onset of straining stimulates the baroreceptors leading to peripheral vasoconstriction (208.1).
  d) T At the end of the manoeuvre, as cardiac output is ejected into a constricted circulation, arterial pressure will rise above normal (208.1).
  e) T A working definition of the Valsalva manoeuvre (208.1).

209a) T The original manoeuvre described by Sellick is more generally known as cricoid pressure (209.1).
  b) F Sellick's manoeuvre describes the compression of the oesophagus between cricoid cartilage and vertebral body (209.1).
  c) F If applied correctly some distortion of the glottis will be seen (209.1).
  d) F Vomiting is active. Regurgitation is passive. If cricoid pressure is applied during vomiting there is a risk that oesophageal rupture will occur (209.1).
  e) T Prevention of regurgitation is the purpose of Sellick's manoeuvre (209.1).

210a) T A wide variety of tumours secrete hormones and all these completions are true. Hypercalcaemia may result from secretion of parathyroid hormone (210.1).
  b) T From secretion of ADH (210.1).
  c) T From secretion of ACTH (210.1).
  d) T From secretion of TSH (210.1).
  e) T From secretion of insulin (210.1).

211 Damage to the cauda equina causes:
a) urinary incontinence
b) faecal incontinence
c) impotence
d) sensory loss in the legs
e) abnormal leg reflexes

212 Concerning pulse oximetry:
a) oxyhaemoglobin and deoxyhaemoglobin light absorption is equal at the isobestic point of 660 nm
b) measurements are accurate in the presence of carboxyhaemoglobin
c) measurements are accurate in the presence of high levels of bilirubin
d) measurements are accurate in the presence of pigmented skin
e) saturation of venous blood may be recorded

213 The inguinal canal:
a) extends from the internal ring medially to the external ring laterally
b) is roofed by the inguinal ligament
c) contains the round ligament of the uterus
d) spermatic cord contains the internal and external spermatic arteries
e) spermatic cord contains autonomic nerve fibres

References		
211.1 Synopsis		p 714–715
212.1 CACC 1:2		p 122–123
212.2 Aitkenhead		p 366–367
213.1 Synopsis		p 668–669

211a) F Urinary retention occurs after cauda equina damage. Following spinal anaesthesia most symptoms and signs are temporary but some may be permanent (211.1).
b) T Faecal incontinence occurs (211.1).
c) T Sexual function is lost (211.1).
d) F The sensory loss is in the lumbosacral distribution (211.1).
e) T Abnormal leg reflexes and temporary paralysis of the peroneal nerve may occur (211.1).

212a) F The absorption of light by both types of haemoglobin is equal at the isobestic point but the isobestic point is 805 nm. An oximeter uses two light emitting diodes (LED), one emitting visible red light of 660 nm and one emitting infrared light of 940 nm wavelength (212.1).
b) F Pulse oximeters give inaccurate readings in the presence of pigments such as carboxyhaemoglobin, methaemoglobin and bilirubin (212.2).
c) F See (b) above (212.2).
d) T Pigmentation of the skin does not modify the reading so an oximeter is helpful in Africans and Asians where cyanosis is difficult to detect clinically (212.2).
e) F Software is designed to 'look' for the pulsatile waveform of the arterial pulse and measure the haemoglobin saturation of this pattern (212.2).

213a) F Caution. The internal ring is lateral to the external ring (213.1).
b) F The inguinal ligament is the floor of the inguinal canal. The roof is made of the fibres of the conjoint tendon of the transversus abdominis muscle and the internal oblique (213.1).
c) T The canal contains the spermatic cord in the male and the round ligament of the uterus in the female (213.1).
d) T The spermatic cord consists of the internal and external spermatic arteries, the artery to the vas deferens, the pampiniform plexus of the veins, the lymphatic vessels, the autonomic nerve fibres and the vas deferens (213.1).
e) T See (d) above (213.1).

214 Functions of the lung include:
   a) excretion of halothane
   b) activation of angiotensin II
   c) inactivation of prostaglandins
   d) metabolism of noradrenaline
   e) synthesis of surfactant

215 With respect to humidifiers:
   a) the condenser humidifier gives 90% relative humidity
   b) nebulisers use the Bernoulli principle
   c) ultrasonic humidifiers are gas driven
   d) water baths are most efficient
   e) water intoxication is a risk

216 In a venturi type oxygen mask:
   a) rebreathing occurs
   b) high gas flow is necessary
   c) performance is variable
   d) increased oxygen flow will increase the inspired oxygen percentage
   e) a tight fit is necessary

References	
214.1 Ganong	p 615
215.1 Ward	p 242–247
216.1 Scurr	p 290–294

214a) T All anaesthetic vapours have a route of excretion through the lung. Perhaps this is not worthy of consideration as a true 'function', however.
  b) F The lung converts angiotensin I to angiotensin II (214.1).
  c) F Prostaglandins are synthesised in the lung (214.1).
  d) T All catecholamines are metabolised to a greater or lesser extent (214.1).
  e) T Obvious (214.1).

215a) T Condenser humidifiers are also known as heat/moisture exchange devices. These humidifiers may achieve relative humidity of around 90% (215.1).
  b) T Nebulisers generally utilise the Bernoulli principle in generating a fine mist of particles after impacting a jet of gas loaded with moisture onto a device such as an anvil (215.1).
  c) F Ultrasonic nebulisers are powered by high-frequency electrical resonators which produce sonic bombardment (215.1).
  d) F Water baths are the least efficient. Ultrasonic nebulisers are the most efficient (215.1).
  e) T Water intoxication is a potential risk of any humidification. It is most marked with ultrasonic types which produce very small droplets (215.1).

216a) F Functional apparatus dead space is eliminated by correct flow rates so that rebreathing will not occur (216.1).
  b) T A high flow system with a variable venturi can be used to provide any required mixture without rebreathing (216.1).
  c) F Venturi devices belong to the fixed performance category, in which the inspired concentration is fixed over the range ±1% (216.1).
  d) F Entrainment ratios remain the same with an increase in oxygen supply but there is an increase in total mixture flow (216.1).
  e) F A tight fit is unnecessary in venturi type devices (216.1).

217 With respect to the heart sounds:
   a) the first sound is made by the closure of the aortic and pulmonary valves
   b) the second sound is made by the closure of the tricuspid and mitral valves
   c) a third sound is abnormal
   d) a fourth heart sound is abnormal
   e) the second sound occurs at the end of ventricular systole

218 Cocaine:
   a) is an amide
   b) is a vasoconstrictor
   c) is effective on mucous membranes
   d) causes CNS stimulation
   e) causes miosis

219 Features of Marfan's syndrome include:
   a) aortic stenosis
   b) cataracts
   c) aortic aneurysm
   d) mitral incompetence
   e) tall stature

References	
217.1 Ganong	p 525
218.1 Dundee	p 290
219.1 Souhami	p 93

217a) F The first heart sound (lub) is made by the sudden closure of mitral and tricuspid valves at the beginning of ventricular systole (217.1).
b) F The second heart sound (dup) is caused by the closure of aortic and pulmonary valves at the end of ventricular systole (217.1).
c) F A third heart sound is heard in a proportion of normal young persons (217.1).
d) T The presence of a fourth heart sound is usually (but not always) pathological (217.1).
e) T See (b) above (217.1).

218a) F Cocaine is an ester of benzoic acid (218.1).
b) T Cocaine has marked vasoconstrictor properties which has lead to its popular use prior to surgical ENT procedures (218.1).
c) T Cocaine is effective topically on mucous membranes (218.1).
d) T Initially euphoria occurs followed by tremors and tonic-clonic convulsions (218.1).
e) F Cocaine causes mydriais, the opposite effect to miosis (218.1).

219a) F Marfan's syndrome includes aortic and mitral incompetence. Take care with this completion (219.1).
b) F Lens dislocation is the classic feature seen (219.1).
c) T Aneurysms of the aorta, including dissecting types, are seen (219.1).
d) T See (a) above (219.1).
e) T Tall stature is usual. Other features are high arched palate, hyperextensible joints and a tendency to spontaneous pneumothorax (219.1).

220 Intermittent positive pressure ventilation (IPPV) reduces:
a) compliance
b) right atrial pressure
c) sodium excretion
d) intrapleural pressure
e) cardiac output

221 Rifampicin:
a) may produce red urine
b) must be given in conjunction with another antibiotic
c) has poor intracellular penetration
d) commonly causes skin rashes
e) is hepatotoxic

222 Functional residual capacity (FRC) is reduced by:
a) age
b) artificial ventilation
c) anaesthesia
d) paralysis
e) oxygen

References	
220.1 Synopsis	p 239–241
221.1 Dundee	p 491–492
222.1 Davenport	p 23
222.2 Nunn	p 357

220a) **T** Compliance is reduced by approximately 50% (220.1).
 b) **F** Right atrial pressure is increased with a resulting fall in venous return and cardiac output (220.1).
 c) **T** Retention of sodium occurs in long term IPPV (220.1).
 d) **F** Intrapleural pressure during IPPV rises on inspiration from -5 cmH_2O to $+3$ cmH_2O and falls to -5 cmH_2O on expiration. During spontaneous respiration the pressure varies between -5 cmH_2O and -10 cmH_2O (220.1).
 e) **T** See (b) above (220.1).

221a) **T** Rifampicin may produce a red colour in urine, saliva and tears occasionally (221.1).
 b) **T** Resistant strains readily emerge and rifampicin should be given in conjunction with another agent to minimise this likelihood (221.1).
 c) **F** The intracellular penetration of rifampicin is particularly good (221.1).
 d) **F** Skin rashes occur with use of the drug, but not commonly (221.1).
 e) **T** Monitoring of liver function during treatment is recommended (221.1).

222a) **F** FRC is thought to increase. Physiological dead space to tidal volume ratio increases (222.1).
 b) **T** In the conscious subject, FRC is reduced slightly (222.2).
 c) **T** FRC is reduced by all anaesthetic drugs. The reduction occurs in the first few minutes and may not return to normal for some hours after the end of anaesthesia. Reduction may be of the order of 16–20% (222.2).
 d) **F** The reduction due to anaesthesia is not changed by paralysis (222.2).
 e) **F** Oxygen is not a factor that changes FRC (222.2).

223 Rapid loss of 500 ml blood leads to:
a) reduced baroreceptor discharge
b) increased urine output
c) venoconstriction
d) reduced peripheral resistance
e) a fall in filtration fraction

224 The following drugs are indicated in porphyria:
a) morphine
b) thiopentone
c) methohexitone
d) ketamine
e) etomidate

225 Gelatine solutions:
a) are not antigenic
b) interfere with cross-matching
c) have molecular weights averaging 100 000 Daltons
d) may be urea linked
e) remain in the circulation longer than dextrans

References	
223.1 Ganong	p 589
224.1 Synopsis	p 393–394
225.1 Dundee	p 552

223a) T Arterial baroreceptors are stretched to a lesser degree and their discharge falls (223.1).
  b) F Afferent and efferent arterioles in the kidney are constricted in response to haemorrhage (500 ml represents 10% loss). Glomerular filtration is depressed but renal plasma flow is reduced even more and thus filtration fraction (GFR/RPF) falls (223.1).
  c) T Vasoconstriction is marked and widespread in both venous and arterial systems (223.1).
  d) F Peripheral resistance rises as a direct consequence of reflex vasoconstriction (223.1).
  e) T See (b) above (223.1).

224a) T Both morphine and pethidine are widely advocated as safe to use in porphyric states (224.1).
  b) F Barbiturates stimulate delta-ALA-synthetase and must therefore be avoided completely (224.1).
  c) F Methohexitone is a barbiturate. The above statements thus apply (224.1).
  d) T Ketamine is said to be a safe induction agent to use in porphyria (224.1).
  e) T Etomidate is probably the agent of choice for induction (224.1). Note that some animal studies have questioned the safety of etomidate in porphyria. Human data is scarce.

225a) F Gelatine solutions belong to three groups: oxypolygelatines, modified fluid gelatine and urea-linked gelatines. All are antigenic with an incidence of anaphylactoid reactions similar to that for dextrans (0.008%) (225.1).
  b) F Cross-matching difficulty is a problem of the dextrans (225.1).
  c) F The gelatin family molecular weights lie in the range 30 000–35 000 Daltons (225.1).
  d) T One of the most commonly used gelatines – Haemacell® – is urea-linked polygelatine (225.1).
  e) F The gelatines are shorter lived in the circulation than are the dextrans (225.1).

226 In the normal kidney:
  a) GFR is the same as RPF
  b) RPF is 125 ml/min
  c) GFR is 600 ml/min
  d) filtration fraction is 0.25
  e) GFR may be measured using inulin

227 On changing from supine to erect:
  a) peripheral resistance falls
  b) heart rate rises
  c) cardiac output falls
  d) compensation mechanisms result from stimulation of receptors in the carotid body
  e) aldosterone secretion increases

228 Aspirin:
  a) inhibits cyclo-oxygenase
  b) reduces body temperature
  c) has a peripheral site of action
  d) accelerates prostaglandin synthesis
  e) is acetyl-salicylic acid

References		
226.1 Ganong		p 655–658
227.1 Ganong		p 583–584
228.1 Dundee		p 231–232

226a) F GFR is glomerular filtration rate, and is a measure of filtration through the glomeruli in the absence of secretion and reabsorption. RPF is renal plasma flow, which represents the amount of plasma filtered by the kidney (226.1).

b) F GFR in the normal kidney is around 125 ml/min. RPF is 625 ml/min or thereabouts (226.1).

c) F See above (b) (226.1).

d) F Filtration fraction is the ratio of GFR to RPF. Normally this lies in the range 0.16–0.20 (226.1).

e) T Measurement of GFR requires a substance that is neither reabsorbed nor secreted in the tubules. Inulin (a high molecular weight polymer of fructose) meets these criteria (226.1).

227a) F One of the compensatory mechanisms which comes into play is arteriolar vasoconstriction which increases peripheral vascular resistance and maintains the blood pressure (227.1).

b) T Tachycardia compensates to some extent for the fall in venous return (227.1).

c) T Cardiac output falls due to reduced preload (227.1).

d) F The baroreceptors induce the compensatory response. They are located in the carotid <u>sinus</u>, not the carotid body (227.1).

e) T Secretion of both aldosterone and renin is enhanced (227.1).

228a) T Aspirin inhibits cyclo-oxygenase, an enzyme which is responsible for the conversion of arachidonic acid to PGG_2 and PGH_2 (228.1).

b) F Aspirin has no effect on normal temperature. It will reduce pyrexia, however, and in toxic doses hyperpyrexia is induced (228.1).

c) T The available evidence suggests that this is so (228.1).

d) F Prostaglandin synthesis is inhibited, as is release (228.1).

e) T Aspirin is acetyl-salicylic acid, originally obtained from willow bark (228.1).

229 The following drugs are protein bound:
a) thiopentone
b) aspirin
c) warfarin
d) halothane
e) ketorolac

230 Hypoxia following laparotomy may be due to:
a) overtransfusion of crystalloid
b) reduced FRC
c) reduced closing capacity
d) upper abdominal surgery
e) dehydration

231 With respect to capnography:
a) confirmation of ETT placement is possible
b) a fall in $P_{ET}co_2$ may be due to rebreathing
c) a fall in $P_{ET}co_2$ implies pulmonary embolism
d) it may be used as a ventilator alarm
e) it is unsuitable for use in a circle system

References	
229.1 Dundee	p 142–143
229.2 Dundee	p 238
229.3 Dundee	p 40
229.4 Dundee	p 98–99
229.5 Data Sheet	p 1682
230.1 CACC 2:1	p 8–13
231.1 CACC 1:3	p 179–180

229a) T Thiopentone is 65–85% protein bound; the binding is dependent on pH (229.1).
b) T Aspirin is 80–90% protein bound, mainly to albumin (229.2).
c) T Warfarin and diazepam are very highly protein bound at 98–99%, mainly to albumin (229.3).
d) F Halothane is not bound to protein but dissolves in solution and is more soluble in fat than in blood (229.4).
e) T Ketorolac is over 99% protein bound (229.5).

230a) T Pulmonary oedema will occur with overtransfusion of crystalloid leading to hypoxia and respiratory failure (230.1).
b) T There is a marked decrease in FRC for several days post-operatively following upper abdominal surgery (230.1).
c) F Closing capacity is the lung capacity at which the alveoli start to collapse because of surrounding forces on the lung. Closing capacity is either unchanged or increased (230.1).
d) T Pulmonary changes are minimal with <u>lower</u> abdominal surgery. The size and position of the incision is important. Small incisions impede lung function less than large incisions, and a subcostal incision is less of a disturbance than midline incisions (230.1).
e) T Thick tenacious sputum with plugging occurs secondary to dehydration. Hypoxia leads to increased risk of pneumonia (230.1).

231a) T On condition that the waveform of ventilation is also inspected. The stomach can contain gas in equilibrium with the tissues so the stomach may provide CO_2 at a waning $P_{ET}co_2$ for the first few breaths on oesophageal intubation (231.1).
b) F In rebreathing, end tidal CO_2 ($P_{ET}co_2$) rises together with $Paco_2$. There is an elevated plateau and an increased inspiratory CO_2 tension ($P_{I}co_2$) (231.1).
c) T A pulmonary embolus results in a sudden increase in alveolar dead space; gas from this area dilutes the CO_2 from perfused alveoli with a resultant, sudden reduction in $P_{ET}co_2$ (231.1).
d) T A capnograph can be used as an apnoea alarm and a disconnection alarm (231.1).
e) F The capnograph <u>should</u> be used in circle systems to monitor the function of the soda lime; in very low flow systems it may be desirable to return the sampled gas to the circle (231.1).

232 The partial pressure of a volatile agent in the brain is dependent on:
a) alveolar ventilation
b) concentration of the agent in expired gas
c) transfer across the alveoli
d) cardiac output
e) solubility

233 In the normal lung:
a) There are 30 airway generations
b) vital capacity is the largest amount of air that can be expired after maximal inspiration
c) the diaphragm accounts for 50% of the change in intrathoracic volume during quiet breathing
d) surfactant is produced by type I pneumocytes
e) hysteresis is seen

234 Surgical diathermy:
a) commonly delivers 1 kW of power
b) operates at frequencies around 10 kHz
c) requires good contact of the indifferent electrode
d) may be unipolar or bipolar
e) may be safely used on patients having cardiac pacemakers

References	
232.1 Dundee	p 97–100
233.1 Ganong	p 599–609
234.1 Ward	p 334–337

232a) T The partial pressure may also be referred to as tension. The tension of a volatile agent in the brain is directly dependent on alveolar ventilation. Put simply, the agent must be transported from the gas mixture to the alveoli and thence into the circulation (232.1).

b) F Concentration in the <u>inspired</u> mixture is the determining feature (232.1).

c) T This should be obvious. Note the comments in (a) above (232.1).

d) T Cardiac output is responsible for transporting the agent from pulmonary circulation to systemic (and thence to the brain). Note the paradoxical situation in shock states, when low cardiac output causes a more rapid rise in equilibration between brain and arterial tensions (232.1).

e) T Solubility of the agent is a determinant of alveolar to blood transfer (232.1).

233a) F There are 23 generations of airways as originally described in a paper by Weibel (233.1).

b) T A working definition of vital capacity (233.1).

c) F The diaphragm accounts for 75% of the change in intrathoracic volume during quiet respiration (233.1).

d) F Surfactant is produced by type II pneumocytes (233.1).

e) T Pressure-volume loops from the normal lung clearly demonstrate hysteresis (233.1).

234a) F The power output of most surgical diathermy machines is of the order of 50–500 W (234.1).

b) F Frequencies are not standardised but most lie in the range 0.5–1.5 mHz (234.1).

c) T Good contact is essential to provide a large surface area. In this way, heating at the indifferent site may be minimised (234.1).

d) T In a bipolar system the current is passed between forcep points. This earth-free system does not require any current to pass through the body but is low powered (234.1).

e) T The limited information which exists suggests that unipolar diathermy inhibits pacemaker potential generation (234.1).

235 In cardiomyopathy:
a) ejection fraction is always small
b) ventricular thickening is a constant feature
c) aetiology includes high alcohol consumption
d) features of several types may coexist
e) prevalence is highest in Europeans

236 Features of Cushing's syndrome include:
a) hypertension
b) anabolism
c) osteoporosis
d) decreased facial hair
e) enlargement of the sella turcica

237 Oxytocin:
a) acts only on the uterus
b) may cause water intoxication
c) is secreted by the anterior lobe of the pituitary gland
d) is active orally
e) relaxes vascular smooth muscle

References	
235.1 Souhami	p 417–419
236.1 Ganong	p 348–349
237.1 Dundee	p 509

235a) F A distinction should be made between the different types of cardiomyopathy. Dilated, hypertrophic and restrictive types have different features. Although the ejection fraction is small in dilated cardiomyopathy, it is large in HOCM (hypertrophic cardiomyopathy) and well maintained in restrictive cardiomyopathy (235.1).
  b) F Ventricular thickening is seen in HOCM and restrictive types, <u>not</u> dilated cardiomyopathy (235.1).
  c) T Amongst many other causes (235.1).
  d) T Clinical features of more than one type of cardiomyopathy may co-exist (235.1).
  e) F The highest race prevalence occurs in Africans but the reason for this is not clear (235.1).

236a) T Hypertension is common. It occurs in 85% of sufferers either from increased secretion of deoxycorticosterone, angiotensinogen or due to a direct vascular effect (236.1).
  b) F Protein catabolism is the rule leading to protein depletion (236.1).
  c) T Bone formation is reduced and resorption is increased (236.1).
  d) F Facial hair is increased and acne common. These are effects which result from increased secretion of adrenal androgens (236.1).
  e) T The sella turcica is not always enlarged. Small adenomas, for example, may not result in X-ray changes of the pituitary region (236.1).

237a) F Oxytocin has effects on the breasts and vascular system, amongst others (237.1).
  b) T The close structural resemblance of the molecule to ADH is responsible for this effect (237.1).
  c) F Oxytocin is secreted by the posterior lobe of the pituitary (237.1).
  d) F Oxytocin must be given by intravenous infusion (237.1).
  e) T Although transient, the effect on vascular smooth muscle is marked (237.1).

238 The sodium concentration in the following fluids is less than 50 mmol/l:
a) saliva
b) sweat
c) CSF
d) urine
e) bile

239 Features of an ideal inhalational agent include:
a) flammability
b) high solubility
c) chemical stability
d) analgesia
e) volatility

240 The metabolic response to injury:
a) induces hypoglycaemia
b) causes increased urine output
c) results in increased potassium excretion
d) results in increased sodium excretion
e) lasts 24 hours

References	
238.1 Dunnill	p 155
239.1 Review 3	p 110–119
240.1 Synopsis 10e	p 749

238a) F Saliva contains 112 mmol/l sodium (238.1).
   b) F Sweat contains 50 mmol/l sodium (238.1).
   c) F CSF sodium concentration is 140 mmol/l (238.1).
   d) F Urine contains around 70 mmol/l sodium (238.1).
   e) F Bile contains 140 mmol/l sodium (238.1).

239a) F The ideal inhalational anaesthetic agent should be non-flammable in the range of concentrations used in clinical practice (239.1).
   b) F Optimum solubility is low. This yields the advantage of quick onset of action, as equilibration of alveolar tension with neurolipid is easily attained (239.1).
   c) T Good in-vitro stability is desirable. This will give good shelf life. Stability in the presence of soda lime is also desirable (239.1).
   d) T Analgesia is desirable. Most agents in use currently do not possess this property although some older agents were good analgesics (for example diethyl ether) (239.1).
   e) T Obvious! (239.1).

240a) F The metabolic response to injury is seen after surgical procedures. Commonly, hyperglycaemia is seen as steroid output rises (240.1).
   b) F Water retention occurs for 24–36 h. Urine output is reduced (240.1).
   c) T Potassium excretion is increased with maximum excretion occurring at 24 h (240.1).
   d) F Sodium retention is impaired for 4–6 days independent of intake (240.1).
   e) F The response may last six days or so (240.1).

241 Myasthenia gravis:
a) is a disease of fatiguable weakness in smooth muscle
b) is more common in men
c) is associated with thymoma
d) is associated with thyrotoxicosis
e) results in raised antibody titres to acetylcholine receptors

242 The following effects apply to acetazolamide:
a) carbonic anhydrase inhibition
b) urinary acidification
c) nephrocalcinosis
d) metabolic alkalosis
e) raised intra-ocular pressure

243 In Raynaud's phenomenon:
a) venous spasm occurs
b) attacks are precipitated by motion
c) associated collagen diseases are common
d) attacks may be random
e) it is commoner in the elderly

References	
241.1 Souhami	p 946–947
242.1 Dundee	p 466–467
243.1 Souhami	p 448–449

241a) F Myasthenia gravis is a condition characterised by fatiguable weakness of <u>striated</u> muscle (241.1).
   b) F Women sufferers outnumber men by 2 to 1. Onset of the disease is usually in early adult life. Neonatal myasthenia is seen in babies of affected mothers (241.1).
   c) T The association with thymoma is well documented. The thymic histology usually shows hyperplasia (241.1).
   d) T Myasthenia gravis is associated with thymoma, thyrotoxicosis, diabetes mellitus and rheumatoid arthritis, which probably reflects an auto-immune aetiology (241.1).
   e) T Approximately 90% of patients have elevated titres of antibodies to acetylcholine receptors (241.1).

242a) T Carbonic anhydrase is inhibited in the proximal tubule. The main therapeutic use for acetazolamide is not, however, as a diuretic (the effect is only mild) but as a reducer of intra-ocular pressure (242.1).
   b) F The urine is rendered alkaline as acetazolamide limits the availability of hydrogen ions for excretion (242.1).
   c) T Long-term treatment may result in renal calculi and the development of nephrocalcinosis (242.1).
   d) F Alkaline urine output eventually leads to metabolic acidosis (242.1).
   e) F See (a) above (242.1).

243a) F Raynaud's disease is characterised by arteriolar spasm (243.1).
   b) T Attacks of spasm may be triggered by cold, motion or occur at random (243.1).
   c) T A point of semantics. Raynaud's phenomenon is the term applied when there is an association with collagen disease and skin changes. It is otherwise termed Raynaud's <u>Syndrome</u> (243.1).
   d) T See (b) above (243.1).
   e) F The incidence is higher in young women (243.1).

244 Pain on injection is associated with:
a) thiopentone
b) methohexitone
c) propofol
d) ketamine
e) etomidate

245 The following are correct:
a) blood filter pore size 40 μm
b) epidural filter pore size 10 μm
c) standard adult giving sets provide 60 drops/ml
d) activated charcoal absorbs nitrous oxide
e) exposure to pollution in the operating theatre is regulated by COSHH

246 In fat embolism:
a) skin signs occur immediately
b) X-ray changes may be seen
c) purpuric rash is common
d) fat may be visible in retinal vessels
e) Pa_{O_2} will be low

References	
244.1 Aitkenhead	p 175–176
245.1 Ward	p 278–298
246.1 Synopsis	p 788

244a) **F** Pain on injection does not occur with thiopentone (provided the injection is not intra-arterial) (244.1). The reference provides a useful comparative table of the properties of the commonly employed induction agents. Note that injection of thiopentone into very small veins may cause discomfort in a small number of patients.

b) **T** Around a quarter of patients receiving methohexitone complain of pain (244.1).

c) **T** The incidence of pain is 40% or so (244.1).

d) **F** Ketamine does not cause pain on injection (244.1).

e) **T** Not only pain, but also thrombophlebitis, is known to result after administration of etomidate. If small veins are used the incidence of pain on injection is 80% (244.1).

245a) **T** Blood filters are usually either screen or depth types. Screen filters are most commonly used (e.g. Pall) and these have a pore size of 40 μm. Some filter types have a pore size of 20 μm (245.1).

b) **F** Filters used in line with epidural catheters are absolute bacterial filters. The pore size is usually 0.5 μm (245.1).

c) **F** Standard giving sets provide 15-20 drops/ml. Paediatric giving sets provide 60 drops/ml (245.1).

d) **F** Activated charcoal absorbers (aldasorber) absorb vapours but not nitrous oxide (245.1).

e) **T** COSHH is 'Control of Substances Hazardous to Health', a code of practice operating under the Health and Safety at Work Act. It is recommended that exposure to pollutants in the operating theatre should be controlled to a level to which workers may be exposed day after day without adverse effect on health. No exposure levels have been set (245.1).

246a) **F** Skin changes, usually purpura and petechiae, are usually seen one or two days after the event (246.1).

b) **T** Radiological signs are those of bilateral shadowing (246.1).

c) **T** A purpuric rash and petechiae are common signs (246.1).

d) **T** On opthalmoscopy fat globules may be seen tracking along the retinal vessels. This may be a valuable diagnostic aid (246.1).

e) **T** Shunting means that the low Pao_2 may not respond to increased inspired oxygen concentrations (246.1).

247 The following are complications of supraclavicular brachial plexus block:
a) paralysis of the cervical sympathetic chain
b) chest pain
c) motor block
d) haemorrhage
e) surgical emphysema

248 With regard to the diaphragm:
a) the right crus arises from L1, 2 and 3
b) the IVC pierces the diaphragm at the level of T6
c) the phrenic nerves pierce the muscular part of the diaphragm
d) the sympathetic chain passes under the arcuate ligaments
e) it has a central fibrous tendon continuous with the fibrous pericardium

249 Gastric acid secretion:
a) increases gastric emptying
b) is stimulated by histamine
c) is stimulated by gastrin secretion
d) is achieved by parietal cells
e) is abolished by vagotomy

References	
247.1 Synopsis	p 642–648
248.1 Gray's	p 592–593
249.1 Berne	p 670
249.1 Ganong	p 459

247a) T Horner's syndrome results from paralysis of the cervical sympathetic chain. It is a frequent accompaniment to the supraclavicular approach to the brachial plexus (247.1).
b) T Chest pain may occur due to either irritation of the nerve to serratus anterior or pneumothorax (247.1).
c) T Motor blockade is inevitable and leads to a useless limb for the duration (247.1).
d) T Puncture of vessels, particularly the subclavian artery, may lead to haematoma formation (which is usually harmless) (247.1).
e) T Pneumothorax may result because the apical dome of the pleura is underlying Sibson's fascia and may be pierced by the needle. Surgical emphysema will follow (247.1).

248a) T The right crus arises from L1, 2, 3 and the left crus from L1 and 2 only (248.1).
b) F The level of penetration of the IVC is T8–9 (248.1).
c) F Caution! The left phrenic nerve pierces the dome of the diaphragm, which is muscular. The right phrenic nerve pierces the central tendon in close relation to the IVC. The correct answer here is therefore 'false'.
d) T The sympathetic ganglionated trunks lie behind the medial arcuate ligaments (248.1).
e) T The central tendon is a fibrous plane that merges with the fibrous pericardium (248.1).

249a) F This is a notoriously ambiguous completion. Gastric acid secretion is usually mediated via gastrin which tightens the pyloric sphincter and inhibits gastric emptying. Gastric acid secretion which reaches the duodenum has a definitive effect to reduce gastric motility. The effect of gastric acid secretion as a sole entity is impossible to assess (249.1).
b) T The effect of exogenous and endogenous histamine is an increase in gastric acid secretion mediated via H_2 receptors (249.1).
c) T The main mechanism of the secretion of gastric acid (249.1).
d) T Parietal cells are responsible for the formation and release of hydrochloric acid (249.1).
e) F Vagotomy removes the nervous stimulation of gastric acid secretion but humoral and local factors remain operative (249.1).

---

250 Which of the following have blood/gas solubility coefficients greater than 2:
a) nitrous oxide
b) halothane
c) enflurane
d) isoflurane
e) diethyl ether

---

251 The following drugs are water soluble:
a) diazepam
b) propofol
c) etomidate
d) ketamine
e) vecuronium

---

252 A spirometer may be used to measure:
a) tidal volume
b) functional residual capacity
c) total lung capacity
d) vital capacity
e) residual volume

References

250.1 Dunnill   p 7

251.1 Dundee   p 186
251.2 Dundee   p 159
251.3 Dundee   p 155
251.4 Dundee   p 165
251.5 Dundee   p 307

252.1 West   p 12–13
252.2 Nunn   p 39
252.3 Synopsis   p 32–33

250a) F The Ostwald solubility coefficient at 37°C for nitrous oxide is 0.47 (250.1).
   b) T 2.5 is the quoted answer (250.1).
   c) F 1.9 is the correct answer. There is no margin of error allowed, so do not guess (250.1).
   d) F The correct answer is 1.4 (250.1).
   e) T The correct answer is 12 (250.1).

251a) F Diazepam is insoluble in water. It is available in an organic solution or an emulsion, for example Intralipid® (251.1).
   b) F Propofol is insoluble in water and although it was originally solubilised in Cremphor EL it is now available dissolved in Intralipid® (251.2).
   c) T Etomidate sulphate is soluble in water but is unstable. Commercially available etomidate is dissolved in a 35% propylene glycol solution and is stable for 2 years (251.3).
   d) T Ketamine is water soluble (251.4).
   e) T Vecuronium dissolves in water but is unstable (it is stable for 24 h at room temperature and several days at 4°C). To achieve stability vecuronium is supplied as a buffered lyophilised cake (251.5).

252a) T The simplest measurement to make with a spirometer is the tidal volume (252.1). It is important to commit a diagram of lung volumes to memory. The referenced diagram does not contain all the possible combinations and terms and may need to be supplemented with others (for example expiratory reserve volume) (252.2, 252.3).
   b) F Functional residual capacity is measured using the helium dilution technique or body plethysmograph (252.1).
   c) F Expiration to a lung volume of zero is not possible. Therefore total lung capacity cannot be measured using a spirometer (252.1).
   d) T A spirometry trace can display vital capacity (252.1).
   e) F Residual volume cannot be measured using spirometry as it would involve expiring to a lung volume of zero (252.1).

253 Dopamine:
a) causes an increase in renal blood flow at 3 μg/kg.min⁻¹
b) causes peripheral vasoconstriction at 7 μg/kg.min⁻¹
c) can be given with 1.4% sodium bicarbonate
d) may cause supraventricular tachyarrhythmias
e) can be given via a peripheral vein

254 Airway resistance may be increased by:
a) atropine
b) intubation
c) reduced functional residual capacity
d) changing from erect to supine
e) morphine

255 500 ml of group A Rhesus positive blood may be given to a female patient of blood group:
a) AB Rhesus negative
b) A Rhesus negative
c) O Rhesus negative
d) O Rhesus positive
e) AB Rhesus positive

References	
253.1 Dundee	p 351–352
254.1 Aitkenhead	p 30
255.1 Aitkenhead	p 133–134

253a) T At levels of 3 μg/kg.min^{-1} or less dopamine will stimulate the dopaminergic (DA) receptors of the kidney. This results in an increase in renal blood flow and glomerular filtration (253.1).
  b) F Between 5 μg/kg.min^{-1} and 10 μg/kg.min^{-1} dopamine stimulates cardiac beta receptors which increases stroke volume and cardiac output. There is little or no effect on the peripheral vascular beds and systemic vascular resistance is unchanged (253.1).
  c) F Alkaline solutions rapidly inactivate dopamine. Dopamine can be diluted in 5% dextrose, 0.9% saline and dextrose saline (253.1).
  d) T In high doses dopamine will cause tachyarrhythmias and there is a high incidence of both supraventricular tachyarrhythmias and ventricular tachyarrhythmias (253.1).
  e) F Dopamine should always be given via a central vein as extravasation from a peripheral vein into subcutaneous tissues may cause sloughing of the skin (253.1).

254a) F Atropine and hyoscine cause bronchodilatation with a resultant increase in anatomical dead space and a decrease in airway resistance (254.1).
  b) T Most of the increase is due to the endotracheal tube itself. The resistance of a tube and connections is of the order of 0.4–0.6 kPa/l.s^{-1} for adults (254.1).
  c) T A reduction in functional residual capacity results in a reduction of the airway calibre and an increase in resistance (254.1).
  d) T On changing from erect to supine functional residual capacity falls and this results in a reduction in airway calibre (254.1).
  e) T Morphine can cause bronchial constriction by release of histamine (254.1).

255a) F When answering this question remember that the stem refers to the donor blood and the completions to the possible recipients. Rhesus negative women of child bearing age will develop antibodies if transfused with Rhesus positive blood; if antibodies to Rhesus antigens are already present then a transfusion reaction may occur. Transfused cells will be rapidly destroyed even in the absence of a reaction. Antibodies will be formed if they were not present and a future Rhesus positive foetus will become a problem (255.1).
  b) F The important feature is the Rhesus negative female patient (255.1).
  c) F The important feature is the Rhesus negative female patient (255.1).
  d) F Group O blood contains anti-A and anti-B antibodies (255.1).
  e) T Group AB is sometimes called the 'universal recipient' and the Rhesus group is also compatible (255.1).

256 Anatomical dead space:
a) increases when supine
b) increases with neck flexion
c) does not change with tidal volume
d) is increased by atropine
e) increases with paralysis and IPPV

257 The following white cell counts are correct:
a) neutrophils $0.2 \times 10^9/l$
b) monocytes $3 \times 10^9/l$
c) lymphocytes $3 \times 10^9/l$
d) basophils $2 \times 10^9/l$
e) eosinophils $0.4 \times 10^9/l$

258 Spontaneous hyperventilation may lead to:
a) increased cerebral blood flow
b) increased alveolar P_{O_2}
c) hypocapnia
d) decreased total plasma calcium
e) shift to the right of the oxygen dissociation curve

References	
256.1 Aitkenhead	p 30
257.1 Dunnill	p 77
258.1 Ganong	p 642
258.2 Synopsis 10e	p 78–79

256a) F Anatomical dead space is greatest in the standing position and least in the supine position (256.1).
  b) F Anatomical dead space is greatest with the neck extended and least with the neck flexed (256.1).
  c) F There is a direct relationship between tidal volume and anatomical dead space (256.1).
  d) T Atropine has a bronchodilator effect and it is this which accounts for the increase in anatomical dead space (256.1).
  e) T There is some controversy over the issue. It is thought that paralysis and IPPV cause some increase in anatomical dead space per se (256.1).

257a) F The normal neutrophil count is $2.5-7.5 \times 10^9/l$. This is 40–75% on differential. All the differential counts will be found in the reference (257.1).
  b) F The normal monocyte count is $0.2-0.8 \times 10^9/l$.
  c) T The range extends between $1.5-3.5 \times 10^9/l$.
  d) F The normal basophil count is $0-0.1 \times 10^9/l$.
  e) T The normal range is $0.04-0.44 \times 10^9/l$.

258a) F Spontaneous hyperventilation leads to hypocapnia which is a potent cerebral vasoconstrictor. Thus cerebral blood flow falls (258.1).
  b) F Alveolar Po_2 falls. This is due to the periodic breathing which develops from excessive carbon dioxide washout (258.1).
  c) T Obvious and logical (258.1).
  d) F With the development of respiratory alkalosis comes a fall in ionised calcium but a small rise in total plasma calcium (258.2).
  e) F The oxygen dissociation curve is shifted to the left (258.2).

259 Flow can be measured by:
a) the Fick principle
b) high frequency sound wave reflection
c) Wheatstone bridge
d) pressure drop across a constriction
e) Coanda effect

260 The following are correct values for arterial blood:
a) Pa_{O_2} 10 kPa
b) pH 7.4
c) Hydrogen ion concentration 20 nmol/l
d) standard bicarbonate 30 mmol/l
e) P_{CO_2} 7 kPa

261 The following facts are true of nitrous oxide:
a) the velocity of sound is faster than in oxygen
b) it is flammable
c) molecular weight 44 Daltons
d) specific gravity 2
e) critical temperature 71°C

References	
259.1 Parbrook	p 42–43
259.2 Parbrook	p 162–165
259.3 Parbrook	p 183
259.4 Parbrook	p 24–27
259.5 Parbrook	p 38–39
259.6 Parbrook	p 27–28
260.1 Dunnill	p 73–75
261.1 Synopsis	p 132–137

259a) T An example of the application of the Fick principle is the measurement of blood flow through the lungs by oxygen uptake or carbon dioxide excretion (259.1).

b) T The Doppler effect is utilised in the ultrasonic detection of blood flow. This effect is experienced as the change in pitch of sound as a rapidly moving vehicle passes the observer (259.2).

c) F A Wheatstone bridge is used to measure electrical resistance (259.3).

d) T A tube with a constriction is a venturi and the fall in pressure at the constriction, which is proportional to flow, is called the Bernoulli effect (259.4). These terms are often used in relation to nebulisers and entrainment devices (259.5).

e) F The Coanda effect relates to streams of fluid clinging to the walls of tubes and is the principle upon which fluidic valves work (259.6).

260a) F Although 10 kPa is a reasonable working figure in elderly patients, the quoted normal values are 12–15 kPa (260.1).

b) T Normal pH range is 7.36–7.45 (260.1).

c) F Hydrogen ion concentration is the SI unit applied to acid-base status. The normal arterial range is 36–44 nmol/l (260.1).

d) F The normal range for <u>standard</u> bicarbonate is 21-25 mmol/l but be careful because the normal range for <u>actual</u> bicarbonate is 24-32 mmol/l (260.1).

e) F Normal range is 4.5–6.1 kPa (260.1).

261a) F The velocity of sound in nitrous oxide is 262 m/s and in oxygen 317 m/s. This is relevant to the differentiation between the two gases using a whistle (unless you are tone deaf) (261.1).

b) F Nitrous oxide is neither flammable nor explosive but can support the combustion of other agents in the absence of oxygen (261.1).

c) T The molecular weight is 44 Daltons (261.1).

d) F The specific gravity is 1.5 so nitrous oxide will sink in air (261.1).

e) F The critical temperature is 36.5°C, the critical pressure is 71.7 atmospheres (261.1).

262 The femoral nerve:
a) is the motor nerve to quadriceps femoris
b) arises from the posterior divisions of L3, L4 and L5
c) supplies the skin of the anterolateral aspect of the thigh
d) is lateral to the femoral artery
e) enters the thigh behind the inguinal ligament

263 With respect to the larynx:
a) the recurrent laryngeal nerve is sensory to the mucosa above the cords
b) the external laryngeal nerve supplies the cricothyroid muscle
c) the recurrent laryngeal nerve carries abductor and adductor fibres
d) the blood supply arises from branches of the superior and inferior thyroid arteries
e) single cord paralysis requires surgery

264 Damage to the following nerves can occur with incorrect positioning in the lithotomy position:
a) sciatic
b) lateral popliteal
c) saphenous
d) obturator
e) femoral

References	
262.1 Synopsis	p 673–675
263.1 Synopsis	p 22
264.1 Synopsis	p 278–279

262a) T The femoral nerve is the motor nerve to quadriceps femoris, sartorius and pectineus (262.1), hence the inability to straight leg raise with an effective femoral nerve block.

b) F It arises from the posterior divisions of L2, L3 and L4 (262.1).

c) F The lateral cutaneous nerve of the thigh supplies the anterolateral aspect of the thigh as far as the knee anteriorly (262.1).

d) T The femoral nerve is lateral to the femoral artery and is separated from the artery by a slip of psoas major at the level of the inguinal ligament (262.1).

e) T The femoral nerve emerges from psoas major, passes between psoas major and the iliacus and enters the thigh behind the inguinal ligament (262.1).

263a) F As well as providing the motor supply to most of the laryngeal muscles, the recurrent laryngeal nerve supplies sensory fibres to the mucosa below the vocal cords (263.1).

b) T The external laryngeal nerve provides the motor supply to cricothyroid and the inferior constrictor of the pharynx (263.1).

c) T There are both abductor and adductor fibres to the vocal cords running in the recurrent laryngeal nerve (263.1).

d) T The arteries run in accompaniment with the superior and inferior laryngeal nerves (263.1).

e) F Paralysis of one cord is often symptomless. In contrast paralysis of both leaves the cords in adduction due to the unopposed action of cricothyroid and this requires surgery (263.1).

264a) F The sciatic nerve can be traumatised by intramuscular injection. Lithotomy position is not quoted as a cause (264.1).

b) T Compression between the head of the fibula and the lithotomy pole can cause damage to the lateral popliteal nerve. Foot drop may result (264.1).

c) T When the leg is supported lateral to the lithotomy pole the saphenous nerve may be trapped between the pole and the medial tibial condyle. Sensory loss results along the medial side of the calf (264.1).

d) F The obturator nerve is not commonly damaged (264.1).

e) F Lithotomy position is not noted for damaging the femoral nerve but the nerve can be damaged by retractors during lower abdominal surgery (264.1).

265 In acclimatisation to altitude:
a) respiratory acidosis occurs
b) red cell 2,3-DPG levels fall
c) ventilation is increased
d) erythropoeitin secretion rises
e) haematocrit rises

266 Stellate ganglion block may produce:
a) exopthalmos
b) perforation of the oesophagus
c) pneumothorax
d) mydriasis
e) lacrimation

267 Digoxin toxicity may produce:
a) nausea and vomiting
b) abdominal pain
c) visual disturbance
d) A-V block
e) tachycardia

References	
265.1 Ganong	p 637–638
266.1 Synopsis	p 639
267.1 BNF	s 2.1.1

265a) F In acclimatisation to altitude hyperventilation develops. This causes a respiratory alkalosis in the early stages (265.1).
   b) F The oxygen haemoglobin dissociation curve is shifted to the left and an accompanying increase in red cell 2,3-DPG decreases the oxygen affinity of haemoglobin. Overall P_{50} is increased (265.1).
   c) T Initial response is small but over three or four days there is a progressive increase in ventilation (265.1).
   d) T Erythropoeitin secretion promptly increases on ascent. This leads to an increase in red cell numbers (265.1).
   e) T See (d) above (265.1).

266a) F The stellate ganglion is formed by the fusion of the last three cervical ganglia with the first thoracic. Blockade produces sympathetic ablation of these segments. Enopthalmia and ptosis (and general features of a Horner's syndrome) follow (266.1).
   b) T One of the complications of the technique. For detail of the anatomy see reference (266.1).
   c) T The apical pleura is at risk from needle puncture during stellate ganglion block (266.1).
   d) F Miosis will be produced (266.1).
   e) T Lacrimation on the ipsilateral side is a sign of a successful block (266.1).

267a) T Toxicity from the cardiac glycosides produces a wealth of clinical signs and symptoms. Nausea and vomiting are frequent indicators of toxicity (267.1).
   b) T Less frequently abdominal pain occurs with subsequent diagnostic confusion (267.1).
   c) T There are many reported visual disturbances following digoxin toxicity the most common of which is xanthopsia or yellow vision. Other colour derangements of vision also occur (267.1).
   d) T A-V block is predominantly seen when there are underlying problems in the conducting system and when there is co-existing myocardial damage, for example previous myocardial infarction (267.1).
   e) T Although bradycardia is most common, ventricular tachycardias may also present problems in digoxin toxicity (267.1).

268 With regard to oral hypoglycaemic drugs:
   a) biguanides require functioning beta cells
   b) biguanides increase insulin secretion
   c) sulphonylureas require functioning beta cells
   d) sulphonylureas do not cross the placental barrier
   e) metformin may interfere with absorption of vitamin B_{12}

269 The sacrum:
   a) is formed by the fused five sacral vertebrae
   b) articulates with L4
   c) articulates with the coccyx
   d) the sacral canal is continuous with the lumbar vertebral canal
   e) the sacral hiatus is covered by subcutaneous fat and skin

270 With respect to the morphology of the lung:
   a) alveoli are lined by four types of epithelial cells
   b) there are 25 generations of airways
   c) the velocity of air flow is greatest in the small airways
   d) lymphatic channels are not abundant
   e) muscarinic receptors produce brochodilation

References

268.1 Rang   p 506–507

269.1 Synopsis   p 731–732

270.1 Ganong   p 600–602

268a) **F** The action of biguanides remains uncertain but is thought to be based on the liver. Biguanides do not require functioning pancreatic tissue for their effect, in contrast to the sulphonylureas (268.1).

b) **F** Biguanides do not affect insulin secretion. They affect liver cell gluconeogenesis and reduce basal hepatic glucose production. Peripheral effects are those of increasing glucose uptake, an effect which requires insulin (268.1).

c) **T** The action of the sulphonylurea-type agents is the stimulation of pancreatic beta cells to produce insulin (268.1).

d) **F** Sulphonylureas are able to cross the placenta and may cause problems to the newborn infant (268.1).

e) **T** Metformin causes lactic acidosis and gastrointestinal upset. Long term use compromises the absorption of vitamin B_{12} (268.1).

269a) **T** The sacrum is a large triangular bone formed by the fusion of vertebrae S1–S5 (269.1).

b) **F** Superiorly the sacrum articulates with L5 (269.1).

c) **T** Inferiorly the sacrum articulates with the coccyx (269.1).

d) **T** Thus a caudal injection is extradural in nature (269.1).

e) **F** The sacral hiatus is covered in the first instance by the sacro-coccygeal membrane (269.1).

270a) **F** There are two types of epithelial cell, that is, type I and II pneumocytes. Other alveolar cells include macrophages, lympho-cytes, APUD cells and mast cells (270.1).

b) **F** There are 23 generations of airways as described by Weibel (270.1).

c) **F** The velocity of air flow is least in the small airways. This is directly due to the extremely large cross-sectional area compared with that of the trachea and large airways (270.1).

d) **F** Lymphatic channels in the lung are more abundant than in any other organ of the body (270.1).

e) **F** Muscarinic receptors are present in the walls of the bronchi. Stimulation results in bronchoconstriction (270.1).

271 Isoflurane:
   a) is an isomer of halothane
   b) can be used in a halothane vaporiser
   c) has an SVP of 184 mmHg
   d) causes hypotension by myocardial depression
   e) should not be used in Caesarian section

272 SAGM blood:
   a) contains donor plasma
   b) has a higher viscosity than whole blood
   c) has a shelf life of 60 days
   d) PCV is 30%
   e) contains mannitol

273 The blood–brain barrier is:
   a) made up of astrocytes
   b) present in neonates
   c) crossed by atropine
   d) crossed by neostigmine
   e) permeable to dopamine

References	
271.1 Synopsis	p 142–143
271.2 Synopsis	p 135
271.3 Synopsis	p 141
272.1 Synopsis	p 330
273.1 Synopsis	p 10
273.2 Ganong	p 497
273.3 Rang	p 699

271a) F Isoflurane is an isomer of enflurane (271.1).

b) T In theory, as the saturated vapour pressures of halothane and isoflurane are so similar (at 20°C; isoflurane 238 mmHg, halothane 243 mmHg (271.2) the same vaporiser can be used. Crossover of agents in vaporisers is not recommended for safety reasons (271.1).

c) F Isoflurane has an SVP of 238 mmHg at 20°C (271.3). Isomers have the same chemical formula but not necessarily the same physical properties. Enflurane is the agent with SVP 184 mmHg.

d) F Hypotension caused by isoflurane is mainly as a result of the fall in peripheral vascular resistance. The myocardial depression caused by isoflurane is less than that caused by equi-MAC halothane or enflurane (271.1).

e) F Isoflurane is described as suitable for Caesarian section at a concentration of 0.75%. There is a dose-related relaxant effect on the pregnant uterus (271.1).

272a) F In SAGM blood (Saline, Adenine, Glucose, Mannitol) the donor plasma has been removed. The plasma is replaced with 100 ml of fluid containing: sodium chloride 140 mmol/l, adenine 1.5 mmol/l, glucose 50 mmol/l and mannitol 30 mmol/l (272.1).

b) F The viscosity is lower than whole blood as the plasma has been replaced with crystalloid fluid (272.1).

c) F At 4–6°C SAGM blood can be stored for 35 days (272.1).

d) F The PCV (packed cell volume) is 60% (272.1).

e) T Mannitol is the 'M' of SAGM; see (a) (272.1).

273a) F No anatomical structure has been defined as the actual blood–brain barrier (273.1).

b) F The barrier develops during the earlier years of life (273.1). Bile pigments can enter the brain in the neonate and cause kernicterus. The adult's brain is protected by the blood–brain barrier (273.2).

c) T Atropine and hyoscine cross the blood–brain barrier more readily than glycopyrronium (273.1).

d) F Neostigmine does not cross the blood–brain barrier but physostigmine does (273.1).

e) F Dopamine does not cross the blood–brain barrier. Penetration of the blood–brain barrier by dopamine is accomplished by pharmacological manipulation in the treatment of Parkinson's disease (273.3).

274 With respect to antiemetic drugs:
a) ondansetron is a 5-HT$_3$ receptor antagonist
b) hyoscine can be given transdermally
c) ondansetron acts via the chemoreceptor trigger zone
d) metoclopramide increases gastric motility
e) domperidone is a D$_1$ receptor antagonist

275 Cerebrospinal fluid:
a) has a higher protein content than blood
b) contains IgG
c) total volume is 70 ml
d) contains white cells
e) is static within the central nervous system

276 During thiopentone-gas-oxygen-relaxant anaesthesia the following signs indicate a need for more relaxant:
a) sweating
b) rise in blood pressure
c) coughing
d) decreased compliance
e) abdominal wall rigidity

References	
274.1 Rang	p 457–459
275.1 Synopsis	p 8–10
276.1 Synopsis	p 197

274a) T Ondansetron is a recently introduced antiemetic agent which acts as an antagonist at $5HT_3$ receptors (274.1).
  b) T A transdermal preparation of hyoscine is useful in the prevention of motion sickness (274.1).
  c) F The effect of ondansetron is not dependent on the chemoreceptor trigger zone (274.1).
  d) T Metoclopramide has a variety of peripheral actions, one of which is to increase the motility of the stomach. This may enhance its anti-emetic effects (274.1).
  e) F Domperidone is an antagonist at D_2 receptors (274.1).

275a) F The protein content of CSF is considerably lower than that of blood, at 200-400 mg/l (275.1).
  b) F There are no antibodies in CSF (275.1).
  c) F CSF volume is split between half cranial and half spinal. Total volume approximates to 140 ml (275.1).
  d) F There are no white cells in CSF outside of some pathological states (275.1).
  e) F There is a dynamic situation of formation, circulation and drainage of CSF (275.1).

276a) F A distinction must be drawn in this context between the need for paralysis and the need for more opioid to suppress reflex response. Sweating is an indication for more opioid (276.1).
  b) F As above, the need is for greater suppression of reflex response, and further relaxation is not indicated (276.1).
  c) T Coughing in response to an ET tube is an indication of the need for more muscle relaxation (276.1).
  d) T Provided that there is no respiratory obstruction to confuse the picture (276.1).
  e) T Rigidity of the abdominal wall can impede surgery and ventilation. Either way, muscle relaxation is appropriate. This assumes that adequate depth of anaesthesia is being maintained (276.1).

277 In anaesthesia for magnetic resonance imaging (MRI):
a) the ECG is used for monitoring
b) anaesthetic gases must be from cylinder supplies
c) the magnetic field is created by a cathode ray tube
d) personnel must be over 6 m away during imaging
e) ferromagnetic objects are drawn to the machine

278 Considering anaesthesia for ECT:
a) propofol is the best induction agent
b) suxamethonium eliminates the risk of fractures
c) sympathetic stimulation produces bradycardia
d) it is safe within one month of a stroke
e) atropine is normally given pre-induction

279 The following are found in systemic lupus erythematosus (SLE):
a) pericarditis
b) elevation of the diaphragm
c) low ESR
d) high incidence in men
e) Raynaud's phenomenon

References	
277.1 Aitkenhead	p 507–510
278.1 Aitkenhead	p 515–516
279.1 Davidson's	p 788–792

277a) F Conventional ECG monitoring is not possible. Pulse oximetry may be used if the connecting lead is long and the oximeter is out of range of the electromagnetic field (277.1).

b) F On the contrary, molybdenum steel cylinders would be drawn towards the magnetic field, so gas supply is drawn from pipelines (277.1).

c) F The cathode ray tube is used to generate the radiation for computerised tomography (CT). An MRI scanner is made up of a large bore magnet and radio frequency transmitter coil (277.1).

d) F The magnetic field presents no known danger to personnel, who may approach safely. It is important to remember that ferromagnetic items will be drawn to the magnet, and the field may damage electronic equipment such as digital watches (277.1).

e) T See (d) above. The magnetic field is so strong that intracranial vascular clips may be dislodged (277.1).

278a) F Propofol is an unsuitable induction agent for ECT as it shortens the seizure duration which may limit the therapeutic nature of the treatment (278.1).

b) T The use of muscle relaxation is advocated to reduce the risk of fractures. Suxamethonium remains the drug of choice (278.1).

c) F The pattern usually seen is that of parasympathetic stimulation (leading to bradycardia) followed by sympathetic stimulation (278.1).

d) F Cerebral blood flow may increase up to 7 times basal level during ECT, a situation potentially hazardous in recent CVA states (278.1).

e) F The use of atropine is no longer considered necessary (278.1).

279a) T Pericarditis, myocarditis and endocarditis may complicate SLE (279.1).

b) T Progressive elevation of the diaphragm occurs and has been named 'shrinking lung syndrome' (279.1).

c) F The ESR is usually high, especially so when the disease is active (279.1).

d) F The female-to-male ratio of the disease is 9 : 1. There is a particularly high incidence in American black females of 1 in 250 (279.1). The reason for this is unknown.

e) T Raynaud's phenomenon is common in SLE (279.1).

280 Organophosphorous compounds:
a) only cause muscarinic effects
b) may be absorbed through the skin
c) rarely cause CNS effects
d) are anticholinesterases
e) poisoning requires treatment with pralidoxime

281 Sequelae specific to spinal (subarachnoid) anaesthesia include:
a) retention of urine
b) backache
c) aseptic meningitis
d) diplopia
e) anterior spinal artery syndrome

282 Trigeminal neuralgia:
a) always involves the three divisions of the nerve
b) presents as a dull pain
c) may be treated with phenytoin
d) may be triggered by cold
e) is accompanied by motor dysfunction

References	
280.1 Dundee	p 588–589
281.1 Synopsis	p 713–714
282.1 Davidson's	p 839

280a) F Organophosphorous compounds are usually met as insecticides. The whole group are cholinesterase inhibitors and give rise to both nicotinic and muscarinic effects (280.1).
   b) T This group of substances may be absorbed through skin, respiratory and gastro-intestinal tracts (280.1).
   c) F Poisoning results in a wide variety of CNS effects including anxiety, irritability, dizziness and eventually convulsions (280.1).
   d) T Organophosphates phosphorylate the active site of the acetyl-cholinesterase enzyme and form a stable complex (280.1).
   e) T Pralidoxime mesylate regenerates the cholinesterase at the neuromuscular junction. It has no effect at autonomic and CNS sites. After 24 h there will be little effect from treatment (280.1).

281a) F Retention of urine is said to be no more common than after general anaesthesia (281.1). This contrasts to epidural techniques.
   b) F The incidence of backache is very similar in spinal and general anaesthesia groups (281.1).
   c) T Aseptic meningitis is a complication (281.1).
   d) T Diplopia is normally a consequence of external rectus palsy induced by block of the VIth cranial nerve which is known to follow spinal anaesthesia (281.1).
   e) T Fortunately rare. Anterior spinal artery syndrome presents with a lower motor neurone picture in the lower limbs without posterior column involvement (281.1).

282a) F Usually pain starts in divisions II and III first but may later spread to all three (282.1).
   b) F The pain of trigeminal neuralgia is said to be typically lancinating. It is severe and sharp in character (282.1).
   c) T The membrane-stabilising drugs are useful in treatment. Phenytoin and carbamazepine have both enjoyed some success (282.1).
   d) T Triggers to the development of the pain include cold, touching, eating and talking (282.1).
   e) F Usually no motor or sensory dysfunction of the trigeminal nerve is demonstrable (282.1).

283 Blood transfusion:
a) may result in hypokalaemia
b) may result in hypocalcaemia
c) should be warmed to 42°C
d) may result in metabolic alkalosis
e) pH of stored blood is 7.4

284 Atracurium besylate:
a) in solution has pH 3.5
b) causes tachycardia
c) should not be used in myasthenia gravis
d) should not be used in patients with atypical cholinesterase
e) can be used in Caesarian sections

285 In patients with haemoglobinopathy:
a) homozygous thalassaemic blood may contain HbF
b) intubation can be difficult in thalassaemia
c) heterozygous thalassaemic blood may contain HbS
d) thalassaemia occurs in West Africans
e) in thalassaemia the iron of the haem group is in the ferric state

References	
283.1 Synopsis	p 328–335
284.1 Synopsis	p 199
285.1 Synopsis	p 438
285.2 Mason	p 296
285.3 Synopsis	p 388–389

283a) F Stored blood may contain up to 30 mmol/l of potassium as the expiry date approaches. Cardiac arrest has resulted (283.1). Do not confuse the later post-transfusion picture when hypokalaemia can be seen.

b) T Normal adults can metabolise the citrate content of one unit of CPD blood in 5 minutes; if the transfusion is rapid, citrate intoxication may occur causing hypocalcaemia, acidosis, tremors and arrhythmias (283.1).

c) F To prevent hypothermia, transfused blood should be warmed using a thermostatically controlled blood warmer but the temperature should never exceed 40°C (283.1).

d) T Although the pH of stored blood varies between 6.6 and 7.2 (due to accumulation of lactic acid, pyruvic acid, citric acid and a raised $P\text{co}_2$) metabolism of citrate can result in metabolic alkalosis (283.1).

e) F The pH of stored blood varies between 6.6 and 7.2 (283.1).

284a) T The solution has a pH of 3.5 (284.1).

b) F There are no vagolytic effects of atracurium. As a result, a bradycardia may be allowed to occur by the use of atracurium (284.1).

c) F Atracurium is quoted as suitable for use in myasthenia gravis (284.1).

d) F Although metabolism is by Hofmann degradation and alkaline ester hydrolysis in the plasma, atracurium is suitable for patients with atypical cholinesterase (284.1). If hydrolysis by cholinesterase is limited, the Hofmann pathway remains as an alternative route of inactivation.

e) T There is no effective crossing of the placental barrier by atracurium (284.1).

285a) T Homozygous thalassaemic blood contains fetal haemoglobin in place of the absent globin chain (285.1).

b) T Intubation difficulties have been noted due to frontal bossing and maxillary bone enlargement secondary to bone marrow hyperplasia (285.2).

c) T Heterozygous thalassaemic blood may contain HbC, HbE or HbS. HbS may cause sickling problems (285.1).

d) T Thalassaemia occurs in a geographical band from the Mediterranean, through the Middle East and Southern Asia as far as New Guinea. Some West Africans also have thalassaemia (285.3).

e) F The iron of the haem group is not changed in thalassaemia. In methaemoglobinaemia the iron in the haem group is oxidised from ferrous to the ferric state (285.3).

286 Heparin:
a) carries an electropositive charge
b) is a sulphated polypeptide
c) is present with histamine in the mast cell
d) affects thrombin
e) has a half-life of 50 min after injection

287 Vecuronium bromide:
a) is excreted renally
b) is supplied in solution
c) is a monoquaternary compound
d) is acidic in solution
e) is a depolarising muscle relaxant

288 The following are constituents of papaveretum:
a) morphine
b) noscapine
c) thebaine
d) codeine
e) histamine

References	
286.1 Rang	p 387–388
287.1 Dundee	p 306–307
287.2 Synopsis	p 199–200
288.1 Vickers	p 182

286a) **F** Heparin is strongly charged which accounts for some of its anticoagulant effect but this charge is electronegative (286.1).
  b) **F** Heparin is a family of sulphated aminoglycans. These molecules are polysaccharides (286.1).
  c) **T** Heparin is found in the mast cell in a complex with histamine (286.1).
  d) **T** The main mechanism of action is the inhibition of antithrombin III which is a naturally occurring inhibitor of thrombin and several other serine proteases (286.1).
  e) **T** The half-life after injection, although dose dependent to some extent, is 40–90 min (286.1).

287a) **T** Renal excretion is only responsible for a small proportion of the excretion. Some 15% is excreted renally in the first 24 h after a dose (287.1).
  b) **F** Vecuronium is supplied as a lyophilised buffered cake which requires reconstitution with water before use (287.1).
  c) **T** The molecule has one quaternary group and one tertiary nitrogen group (287.1).
  d) **T** The pH of the reconstituted solution is 4 (287.2).
  e) **F** Elementary knowledge. Vecuronium is a non-depolarising (competitive) muscle relaxant drug (287.1).

288a) **T** Papaveretum is a mixture containing the water-soluble alkaloids of the opium poppy. 50% of the mixture is anhydrous morphine (288.1).
  b) **T** Noscapine has recently come into the spotlight following in-vitro evidence that it increased the incidence of cell polyploidy. Despite the lack of direct relevance to man, the CSM recommended that papaveretum not be given to females of child-bearing age due to its noscapine content. Note that a formulation without noscapine is now available (288.1).
  c) **T** Thebaine is present (288.1).
  d) **T** Codeine is present. Also contained are papaverine and narcotine (288.1).
  e) **F** There is no histamine in the mixture but papaveretum causes histamine release (288.1).

289 In the child (under 10 years old):
a) MAC is 0.8 times adult value
b) resting respiratory rate decreases throughout childhood
c) tidal volume per kg is greater than the adult value
d) the cricoid ring is the narrowest part of the trachea
e) the epiglottis is doubly curved

290 With respect to anticonvulsants:
a) phenytoin metabolism shows saturation kinetics
b) phenytoin is an antiarrhythmic
c) diazepam is a sodium channel blocker
d) ethosuximide is used to treat grand mal epilepsy
e) carbamazepine is derived from a tricyclic antidepressant

291 Verapamil:
a) can be used with digoxin
b) can be used with beta adrenergic antagonists
c) may cause rhythm disturbances
d) has the same dose for intravenous and oral routes
e) may affect glucose tolerance

References	
289.1 Synopsis	p 574–582
290.1 Rang	p 690–696
290.2 Rang	p 334
291.1 Dundee	p 412–413

289a) F MAC is increased in children. It is highest (1.5 times adult MAC) at 1 year of postconceptual age, i.e. 2 months after full term birth! MAC falls throughout childhood to reach adult levels by the mid 20s (289.1).

b) T Resting respiratory rate decreases throughout childhood (289.1).

c) F The tidal volume per kg (7 ml/kg), FRC (30 ml/kg) and dead space (2 ml/kg) are all similar to the adult figures (289.1).

d) T The narrowest part of the trachea is the indistensible cricoid ring in the subglottic region (289.1).

e) T In the child the larynx appears more anterior, the epiglottis is more floppy than in the adult and it is doubly curved (289.1).

290a) T The result of saturation kinetics is that there is a non-linear relationship between daily dose of phenytoin and steady state plasma concentration. Monitoring of plasma levels is essential (290.1).

b) T Phenytoin belongs to class Ib of the Vaughan-Williams classification of antiarrhythmics (290.2).

c) F Diazepam enhances the action of GABA. Phenytoin causes use dependent sodium channel blockade (290.1).

d) F Ethosuximide is used to treat absence seizures (petit mal) and may exacerbate other forms of epilepsy (290.1).

e) T Carbamazepine is chemically derived from a tricyclic antidepressant (290.1).

291a) T Verapamil can be used with digoxin (carefully) if the ventricular response on digoxin is still too rapid (291.1).

b) F Beta-blocking drugs are a contraindication to verapamil therapy (291.1).

c) T In higher doses, rhythm disturbances may occur as a result of the negative inotropic effects of verapamil (291.1).

d) F There is very extensive first pass liver extraction (oral bioavailability of 10–20%). The intravenous dose is 10 mg over 1–2 min versus an oral dose of 40–120 mg 8 hourly (291.1).

e) T Insulin secretion is controlled by the influx of calcium ions, and all calcium antagonists may affect glucose tolerance (291.1).

292 In dystrophia myotonica:
a) inheritance is by a recessive gene
b) there is an association with cataracts
c) non-depolarising relaxants abolish the myotonia
d) response to depolarising relaxants is normal
e) there is an association with cardiomyopathy

293 Myelomatosis (multiple myeloma):
a) is a malignant condition affecting plasma cells
b) may be diagnosed by electrophoresis
c) is common in the young
d) light chain varieties are most frequent
e) may cause Bence-Jones proteinuria

294 The following effects do not apply to pancuronium bromide:
a) histamine release
b) bradycardia
c) biliary excretion
d) steroidal activity
e) spontaneous breakdown

References

292.1 Synopsis p 412–413

293.1 Davidson's p 745

294.1 Dundee p 305–306

292a) F Dystrophia myotonica is a disease of the membranes of muscle fibres which is inherited as an autosomal dominant (292.1).
b) T Cataracts are a frequent finding (292.1).
c) F A characteristic feature of the disease is that non-depolarising relaxants will not necessarily abolish the myotonia (292.1).
d) F Depolarising muscle relaxant drugs are particularly hazardous. There may be a sustained increase in muscle tone so great as to make intubation impossible (292.1).
e) T Both cardiomyopathy and various conduction defects may occur (292.1).

293a) T In malignant situations the plasma cells manufacture the same immunoglobulin with only one type of light chain. The name for this is monoclonal (293.1).
b) T Although strictly speaking this is confirmation of diagnosis, electrophoresis reveals the presence of a paraprotein band (293.1).
c) F The disease is rare below the age of 30 years, after which the incidence rises to a peak between 60–70 years of age (293.1).
d) F The most common types are IgG paraproteins (293.1).
e) T Light chains may appear in the urine as 'Bence-Jones' proteins (293.1).

294a) F Histamine release is not a major feature of pancuronium (it has been called 'minimal') but the propensity of the drug to release histamine lies between curare and vecuronium (294.1). Be especially careful of the negative wording in this stem.
b) T Tachycardia is seen after the administration of pancuronium. Also common is an increase in arterial pressure (294.1).
c) F Biliary excretion is associated with pancuronium. About 10% is excreted in the bile in the first 24 h after dosage (294.1).
d) T Pancuronium has no steroidal activity (294.1).
e) T Atracurium is the only non-depolarising muscle relaxant whose action shows spontaneous reversal (294.1).

295 **The following are clinical features of Addison's disease:**
   a) weight gain
   b) vitiligo
   c) pigmentation
   d) weakness
   e) decreased body hair

296 **Chemoreceptors are found in:**
   a) the aortic arch
   b) the carotid body
   c) the carotid sinus
   d) the CNS
   e) the aortic body

297 **With regard to dantrolene sodium:**
   a) central effects are rare
   b) hepatotoxicity is a risk
   c) smooth muscle is not affected
   d) it may be given orally
   e) the action of the drug is to encourage the release of calcium ions from the sarcoplasmic reticulum

References	
295.1 Davidson's	p 649
296.1 Ganong	p 626–627
296.2 Ganong	p 555
297.1 Calvey	p 289

295a) F The characteristic feature of Addison's disease is weight loss. Weight gain is often seen in Cushing's syndrome (295.1).

b) T 10–20% of sufferers may have vitiligo which is thought to be an auto-immune phenomenon. Beware of confusion with pigmentation which is more commonly seen in Addison's disease (295.1).

c) T The pigmentation is due to high levels of circulating ACTH (295.1).

d) T Weakness is a feature of Addison's. It may be due to a combination of debility and potassium loss (295.1).

e) T Loss of adrenal androgen output leads to diminution of body hair which is especially marked in the female (295.1).

296a) F Chemoreceptor is a term used for those receptors that are stimulated by a change in the chemical composition of their environment. The aortic arch contains baroreceptors (296.1).

b) T The carotid body is located near the carotid bifurcation. It is thought that the chemoreceptors are the type I glomus cells located in this region (296.1).

c) F The carotid sinus is the location of baroreceptors (296.2).

d) T There are chemoreceptors in the medulla oblongata. This group are sensitive to local hydrogen ion concentration and are intimately connected with the chemical control of respiration (296.1).

e) T The aortic bodies contain peripheral chemoreceptors (296.1).

297a) F There are a variety of central effects attributable to dantrolene. These include dizziness, weakness and tiredness (297.1).

b) T Hepatotoxicity is an occasional risk after treatment (297.1).

c) T The contractility of skeletal muscle, but not that of cardiac and smooth types, is reduced by dantrolene (297.1).

d) T Although it is most frequently thought of in anaesthesia as an agent for use intravenously in malignant hyperthermia, dantrolene enjoys popularity as an oral treatment in spastic conditions (297.1).

e) F Dantrolene prevents the release of calcium ions from the sarcoplasmic reticulum. This prevents indirectly the activation of myosin ATPase and muscle contraction (297.1).

298 The following drugs work by enzyme inhibition:
a) enalapril
b) acetazolamide
c) ibuprofen
d) cimetidine
e) allopurinol

299 Tricyclic antidepressants may cause:
a) decreased intracranial amine concentration
b) salivation
c) drowsiness
d) tachycardia
e) convulsions

300 Pharmacogenetic factors are relevant to:
a) suxamethonium apnoea
b) isoniazid polyneuritis
c) porphyria
d) malignant hyperthermia
e) chloramphenicol agranulocytosis

References

298.1 Dundee		p 430
298.2 Dundee		p 466
298.3 Rang		p 282
298.4 Dundee		p 512
298.5 Rang		p 297
299.1 Dundee		p 587
300.1 Dundee		p 22–24
300.2 Rang		p 114–115
300.3 Vickers		p 38–40

298a) F Enalapril is an inactive prodrug. It is hydrolysed after absorption to enalaprilat, which is an inhibitor of angiotensin converting enzyme. Take care (298.1).

b) T Acetazolamide works by inhibition of the enzyme carbonic anhydrase (298.2).

c) T Ibuprofen in common with many NSAIDs inhibits the enzyme arachidonate cyclo-oxygenase, which is responsible for its therapeutic effects (298.3).

d) F Cimetidine acts by a blocking effect at H_2 receptors. It is incidentally an inhibitor of hepatic microsomal enzymes (298.4).

e) T Allopurinol reduces uric acid synthesis by inhibiting xanthine oxidase (298.5).

299a) F The tricyclic antidepressants inhibit the uptake of noradrenaline and during long-term use cause an increase in intracranial amine concentrations (299.1).

b) F Dry mouth is usual due to the anticholinergic effects of the drugs (299.1).

c) T Drowsiness is seen which may be marked in poisoning (299.1).

d) T Tachycardia and major arrhythmias may occur during treatment (299.1).

e) T Convulsions are most likely in situations of accidental or deliberate overdosage with tricyclic antidepressants (299.1).

300a) T Pharmacogenetics relates inherited factors to the unpredictable response to a drug. Suxamethonium apnoea is an inherited condition due to a recessive gene (300.1, 300.2).

b) T Isoniazid elimination depends on acetylation rate. Genetically there are fast and slow acetylators. The development of isoniazid polyneuropathy is higher in slow acetylators (300.2).

c) T Porphyria is one of the better known pharmacogenetically linked disorders (300.1).

d) T The inheritance of MH susceptibility is complicated. There is autosomal dominant inheritance with incomplete penetrance and variable expression. Pharmacogenetics applies, however (300.1).

e) T Although chloramphenicol agranulocytosis might be considered an idiosyncratic reaction, some of these are genetically determined. It is thought that genetic factors apply to this susceptibility. For detail see reference (300.3).

Bibliography

The bibliography provides the key to the shortened references used throughout the book. The shortened title used in the reference box forms the first line of each section below and this is followed by the full reference. A weighting on the value of each source for revision has been given. Thirty two texts have been used with a total of 465 references. In order to give the candidate an idea of priority during revision the number of references to each text is given in brackets preceding the appraisal of each text. Texts to which the Part 1 FRCA candidate should have constant access are marked with an asterisk (*).

*Aitkenhead

Aitkenhead A R, Smith G (eds) 1990 Textbook of anaesthesia, 2nd edn. Churchill Livingstone, Edinburgh
(53)
Purpose written for trainees in their first 1–2 years of practice, and as such a core text for Part 1 revision. The popularity of the textbook is such that every candidate seems to own a copy. It is important to recognise that although the book is very 'readable' some subjects do not receive very comprehensive coverage and it is necessary to refer to other texts.

Berne

Berne R M, Levy N L 1988 Physiology, 2nd edn. The C V Mosby Company, St Louis
(1)
A major physiology text which has been used to augment the role of Ganong and Guyton, which will be the books that most candidates used as undergraduates.

BMJ

Marsden A K Basic life support: revised recommendations of the Resuscitation Council (UK). British Medical Journal 1989 299: 442–445
Chamberlain D A Advanced life support: revised recommendations of the Resuscitation Council (UK). British Medical Journal 1989 299: 446–448
(2)
A specific source of information on cardiopulmonary resuscitation.

BNF

British national formulary 1993 British Medical Association and The Royal Pharmaceutical Society of Great Britain, London
(19)
The BNF is distributed free of charge to practising doctors. It is a useful source of clinical information on all drugs used in this country. Editions are published six monthly so references are made to sections rather than page numbers. The section numbers remain constant to each subject and are given at the top of each page.

CACC

Hutton P, Pollard B J, Aitkenhead A R, Simpson P J, Willatts S M (eds) 1989 Current anaesthesia and critical care. Churchill Livingstone, Edinburgh
(3)
Contains useful reviews by recognised authors on many aspects of anaesthesia. An important source of information which is more up to date than major texts. The series is designed to build into a reference text over a period. Publication is quarterly and each issue is topic related. Recommended highly.

Calvey

Calvey T N, Williams N F 1982 Principles and practice of pharmacology for anaesthetists, 2nd edn. Blackwell Scientific Publications, Oxford
(2)
Aimed at the level of knowledge of pharmacology required for Part 2 FRCA

Data Sheet

ABPI data sheet compendium 1993–4. Datapharm Publications, London
(3)
A collection of data sheets duplicating those found in each box of drugs. The data sheets contain detailed information on each drug. Although revised annually, references to this book are easy to identify as the compendium is thoroughly alphabetically indexed.

Davenport

Davenport H T 1986 Anaesthesia in the elderly. William Heinemann Medical Books, London
(4)
A recommended text that brings together many aspects of anaesthesia in the elderly.

Davidson's

Edwards C R W, Boucher I A D (eds) 1991 Davidson's principles and practice of medicine, 16th edn. Churchill Livingstone, Edinburgh
(17)
Popular and readable with more than sufficient detail for most general medical subjects.

*Dundee

Dundee J, Clarke R, McCaughey W 1991 Clinical anaesthetic pharmacology. Churchill Livingstone, Edinburgh
(83)
A detailed and accessible book with excellent sections on general pharmacology.

Dunnill

Dunnill R P H, Colvin M P 1989 Clinical and resuscitative data, 4th edn. Blackwell Scientific Publications, Oxford
(12)
A pocket book for reference throughout training packed with factual tables and concise data. Many sections of this book are useful in everyday anaesthesia. Highly recommended.

Ganong

Ganong W F 1989 Review of medical physiology, 14th edn. Appleton Lange, London
(26)
Anaesthesia textbooks may be short of information on physiology. Ganong is a standard evergreen physiology source which remains good value.

Gray's

Williams P L, Warwick R, Dyson M, Bannister L H (eds) 1989 Gray's anatomy, 37th edn. Churchill Livingstone, Edinburgh
(4)
Very clear and helpful anatomical descriptions make Gray's suitable for selected reading.

Guyton

Guyton A C 1986 Textbook of medical physiology, 7th edn. W.B.Saunders, Philadelphia
(17)
A useful supplement to Ganong or alternatively a potential main physiology revision text. Guyton is gaining popularity.

Macleod

Munro J, Edwards C 1990 Macleod's clinical examination, 8th edn. Churchill Livingstone, Edinburgh
(1)
This famous textbook will be known to all medical students. It has been used here for a clinically based question on neurology only.

Mason

Mason R A 1990 Anaesthesia databook: a clinical practice compendium. Churchill Livingstone, Edinburgh
(15)
Relevant to the clinical anaesthetist and packed with fact. Slightly marred by the lack of formal index.

Miller

Miller R D (ed) 1990 Anesthesia, 3rd edn. Churchill Livingstone, New York
(1)
An extensive American two volume text. Suited mostly to Part 3 FRCA revision.

Nimmo

Nimmo W S, Smith G 1990 Anaesthesia. Blackwell Scientific Publications, Oxford
(2)
Nimmo and Smith benefits from its British origins. Too extensive for Part 1 FRCA revision but a useful occasional source.

Nunn

Nunn J F 1987 Applied respiratory physiology, 3rd edn. Butterworths, London
(4)
A detailed and comprehensive volume on applied respiratory physiology written by an anaesthetist. Knowledge of this book early in an anaesthetic career would be an advantage.

Parbrook

Parbrook G D, Davis P D, Parbrook E O 1990 Basic physics and measurement in anaesthesia, 3rd edn. Butterworth Heinemann, Oxford
(16)
Renowned for the illustration of physical principles and for relating them to everyday anaesthetic equipment and techniques.

Rang

Rang H P, Dale M M 1991 Pharmacology, 2nd edn. Churchill Livingstone, Edinburgh
(13)
A comprehensive and well laid out textbook of general pharmacology. The purpose of the book is summarised in its own preface 'this book is intended primarily for pre-clinical medical students'. Recommended for general pharmacology revision.

Review

Kaufman L (ed) 1982– Anaesthesia review. Churchill Livingstone, Edinburgh
(2)
This series attempts to bridge the gap between original papers appearing in journals and the subsequent distillation into textbooks. It succeeds in this regard well. Each volume contains detailed reviews on a topic with detailed referencing.

Scurr

Scurr C, Feldman S, Soni N 1990 Scientific foundations of anaesthesia, the basis of intensive care, 4th edn. Heinemann Medical Books, Oxford
(3)
Contains a large amount of information, far beyond the requirements of Part 1 FRCA. Desirable nonetheless for its clear explanations of basic physics and elementary statistics.

Souhami

Souhami R L, Moxham J 1990 Textbook of medicine. Churchill Livingstone, London
(37)
An undergraduate medical book which is useful for revision of general medical topics. Souhami is well laid out and popular amongst undergraduates.

Sykes

Sykes M K, Vickers M D, Hull C J 1991 Principles of measurement and monitoring in anaesthesia and intensive care, 3rd edn. Blackwell Scientific Publications, Oxford
(1)
A valuable source of material concerning physical principles.

*Synopsis

Atkinson R S, Rushman G B, Davies N J H 1993 Lee's synopsis of anaesthesia, 11th edn. Wright, Bristol
(11th edn. 83 10th edn. 10)
Synopsis provides a very good general coverage of anaesthesia with both detailed information and further reference sources to study. The addition of new subjects in the 11th edition with subsequent deletion of some passages has resulted in occasional directed references to the 10th edition which may prove to be a frustration to newcomers in anaesthesia. The good coverage of well referenced subjects at a reasonable price make this book highly recommended.

Vickers

Vickers M D, Morgan M, Spencer P S J 1991 Drugs in anaesthetic practice, 7th edn. Butterworth Heinemann, Oxford.
(7)
A general text on the pharmacology of anaesthetic drugs. Personal preferences dictate which of the anaesthetic pharmacology texts will be purchased by candidates.

Ward

Davey A, Moyle J T B, Ward C S 1992 Ward's anaesthetic equipment, 3rd edn. W B Saunders Co, London
(15)
The only British reference source on anaesthetic equipment. Unfortunately the frontiers of equipment development advance so rapidly that it is difficult for standard textbooks to keep pace. The authors of Ward have improved the 3rd edition substantially.

West

West J B 1990 Respiratory physiology–the essentials, 4th edn. Williams and Wilkins, London
(3)
Simple but readable. West provides an overview of respiratory physiology which is useful for Part 1 FRCA and is published in convenient pocket size format.

Wildsmith

Wildsmith J A W, Armitage E N 1987 Principles and practice of regional anaesthesia. Churchill Livingstone, Edinburgh
(2)
A major text on regional anaesthesia. The UK standard in this particular field.

Zilva

Zilva J F, Pannall P R, Mayne P D 1988 Clinical chemistry in diagnosis and treatment, 5th edn. Edward Arnold, London
(4)
A specialist clinical biochemistry text. A major strength lies in the clinical emphasis placed on biochemical abnormalities.

Index

The numbers given refer to question numbers rather than page numbers. A number without a letter refers to a complete question (stem and five completions) on the subject. A number followed by a letter (a–e) indicates that only that completion refers to the subject.